Pediatric Dermatology PART I

Editor

KELLY M. CORDORO

DERMATOLOGIC CLINICS

www.derm.theclinics.com

Consulting Editor
BRUCE H. THIERS

January 2022 • Volume 40 • Number 1

ELSEVIER

1600 John F. Kennedy Boulevard ● Suite 1800 ● Philadelphia, Pennsylvania, 19103-2899

http://www.theclinics.com

DERMATOLOGIC CLINICS Volume 40, Number 1
January 2022 ISSN 0733-8635, ISBN-13: 978-0-323-89738-9

Editor: Lauren Boyle
Developmental Editor: Karen Justine Solomon

Dermatologic Clinics (ISSN 0733-8635) is published quarterly by Elsevier Inc., 360 Park Avenue South, New York, NY 10010-1710. Months of publication are January, April, July, and October. Business and editorial offices: 1600 John F. Kennedy Blvd., Suite 1800, Philadelphia, PA 19103-2899. Customer service office: 11830 Westline Drive, St. Louis, MO 63146. Periodicals postage paid at New York, NY, and additional mailing offices. Subscription prices are USD 429.00 per year for US individuals, USD 1,035.00 per year for US institutions, USD 469.00 per year for Canadian individuals, USD 1,071.00 per year for Canadian institutions, USD 525.00 per year for international individuals, USD 1,071.00 per year for international institutions, USD 100.00 per year for US students/residents, USD 100.00 per year for Canadian students/residents, and USD 240 per year for international students/residents. International air speed delivery is included in all *Clinics* subscription prices. All prices are subject to change without notice. **POSTMASTER:** Send address changes to *Dermatologic Clinics*, Elsevier Health Sciences Division, Subscription Customer Service, 3251 Riverport Lane, Maryland Heights, MO 63043. **Customer Service: 1-800-654-2452 (U.S. and Canada); 314-447-8871 (outside U.S. and Canada). Fax: 314-447-8029. E-mail: journalscustomerservice-usa@elsevier.com (for print support); journalsonlinesupport-usa@elsevier.com (for online support).**

Reprints. For copies of 100 or more, of articles in this publication, please contact the Commercial Reprints Department, Elsevier Inc., 360 Park Avenue South, New York, New York 10010-1710. Tel.: 212-633-3874; Fax: 212-633-3820; Email: reprints@elsevier.com.

The *Dermatologic Clinics* is covered in *MEDLINE/PubMed (Index Medicus), Current Contents/Clinical Medicine, Excerpta Medica, Chemical Abstracts,* and *ISI/BIOMED.*

Contributors

CONSULTING EDITOR

BRUCE H. THIERS, MD
Professor and Chairman Emeritus, Department
of Dermatology and Dermatologic Surgery,
Medical University of South Carolina,
Charleston, South Carolina, USA

EDITOR

KELLY M. CORDORO, MD
Professor of Dermatology and Pediatrics,
Chief, Division of Pediatric Dermatology,
Fellowship Director, Pediatric Dermatology,
McCalmont Family Endowed Professor in
Pediatric Dermatology, Department of
Dermatology, University of California,
San Francisco, UCSF Benioff Children's
Hospital, San Francisco, San Francisco,
California, USA

AUTHORS

NNENNA G. AGIM, MD
Associate Professor of Dermatology,
The University of Texas Southwestern Medical
Center, Dallas, Texas, USA

MOHAMMED ALBAGHDADI, MPA
Temerty Faculty of Medicine, University of
Toronto, Toronto, Canada

JAMES ANDERSON- VILDÓSOLA, MD
Department of Dermatology, Hospital Infantil
Niño Jesús, Madrid, Spain

FAIZAL Z. ASUMDA, MD
Department of Clinical Genomics, Mayo Clinic,
Rochester, Minnesota, USA

DIANA BARTENSTEIN REUSCH, MD
Harvard Combined Dermatology Residency
Training Program, Boston, Massachusetts,
USA

MICHAEL BARTON, MD
Division of Dermatology, Department of
Pediatrics, University of Washington School of
Medicine, Seattle Children's Hospital, Seattle,
Washington, USA

MARKUS D. BOOS, MD, PhD
Associate Professor of Pediatrics, Division of
Dermatology, Department of Pediatrics,
University of Washington School of Medicine,
Attending Dermatologist, Seattle Children's
Hospital, Seattle, Washington, USA

KEVIN P. BOYD, MD
Department of Dermatology, Mayo Clinic,
Rochester, Minnesota, USA

SARAH J. COATES, MD
Pediatric Dermatology Fellow, Department
of Dermatology, University of California, San
Francisco, San Francisco, California, USA

KELLY M. CORDORO, MD
Professor of Dermatology and Pediatrics,
Chief, Division of Pediatric Dermatology,
Fellowship Director, Pediatric Dermatology,
McCalmont Family Endowed Professor in
Pediatric Dermatology, Department of
Dermatology, University of California,
San Francisco, UCSF Benioff Children's
Hospital, San Francisco, San Francisco,
California, USA

MARIA C. GARZON, MD
Professor of Dermatology and Pediatrics at
CUMC, Departments of Dermatology and
Pediatrics, Vagelos College of Physicians &
Surgeons, Columbia University Medical
Center, New York, New York, USA

JENNIFER L. HAND, MD
Departments of Dermatology, Clinical
Genomics, and Pediatric and Adolescent
Medicine, Mayo Clinic, Rochester, Minnesota,
USA

ELENA B. HAWRYLUK, MD, PhD
Associate Professor of Dermatology,
Dermatology Section, Department of
Dermatology, Harvard Medical School,
Massachusetts General Hospital, Boston
Children's Hospital, Boston, Massachusetts,
USA

CANDRICE R. HEATH, MD
Assistant Professor of Dermatology, Lewis
Katz School of Medicine, Temple University,
Philadelphia, Pennsylvania, USA

ÁNGELA HERNÁNDEZ-MARTÍN, MD
Department of Dermatology, Hospital Infantil
Niño Jesús, Madrid, Spain

IRENE LARA-CORRALES, MD, MSc
Staff Physician, Pediatric Dermatology, Staff
Pediatric Dermatologist, Division of
Dermatology, Pediatric Dermatology
Fellowship Director, Hospital for Sick Children,
Associate Professor of Pediatrics, University of
Toronto, Toronto, Ontario, Canada

MARY E. LOHMAN, MD
Micrographic Surgery and Dermatologic
Oncology Fellow, Mayo Clinic, Rochester,
Minnesota, USA

TIMOTHY H. McCALMONT, MD
Professor of Pathology and Dermatology,
Co-Director of the UCSF Dermatopathology
and Oral Pathology Service, Departments of
Dermatology and Pathology, University of
California, San Francisco, San Francisco,
California, USA

KIMBERLY D. MOREL, MD
Associate Professor of Dermatology and
Pediatrics at CUMC, Departments of
Dermatology and Pediatrics, Vagelos College
of Physicians & Surgeons, Columbia University
Medical Center, New York, New York, USA

ALEXANDRA J. MORQUETTE, BA
Medical Student, Lewis Katz School of
Medicine, Temple University, Philadelphia,
Pennsylvania, USA

UCHENNA K. OKOJI, MPH
Drexel University College of Medicine,
Philadelphia, Pennsylvania, USA

MARY D. SUN, BSE, BA
Research Fellow, Icahn School of Medicine at
Mount Sinai, New York, USA

MY LINH THIBODEAU, MD, MSc
Staff Clinical Geneticist, Division of Clinical and
Metabolic Genetics, Hospital for Sick Children,
Associate Professor of Pediatrics, University of
Toronto, Toronto, Canada

JAMES TREAT, MD, FAAD
Professor of Clinical Pediatrics and
Dermatology, Perelman School of Medicine at
the University of Pennsylvania, Philadelphia,
Pennsylvania, USA

ANDREA R. WALDMAN, MD
Assistant Professor of Dermatology and
Pediatrics at Mount Sinai Icahn School of
Medicine, New York, New York, USA

Contents

existing data regarding pediatric melanonychia striata and offer an evidence-based approach to its evaluation and management.

Melanocytic nevi are congenital or acquired benign melanocytic neoplasms. The reason for the appearance of melanocytic nevi is not precisely known. Melanocytic nevi frequently occur in children, constituting a common reason for consultation in pediatric dermatology clinics. In our experience, many parents and caregivers present doubts and fears based more on popular beliefs than on data with valid scientific evidence. This review answers their frequently asked questions, such as the risk of malignancy, the importance of nevi location, the warning signs of malignant transformation, best prevention strategies, and optimal management, based on the most recent scientific evidence available.

This article reviews the clinical findings of epidermal nevi and their associated syndromes and provides an update on their pathogenic genetic changes as well as targeted therapies detailed to date.

The understanding of melanocytes biology is fundamental to the study of dermatology. These dendritic cells underly the most feared primary cutaneous malignancy, fuel escalating progress in related immunotherapy, and invariably underlie entire socioeconomic constructs consciously or unconsciously based on skin tone. Various ethno-genotypes combine with increasing frequency over time, increasing the diversity of skin types that may present with dermatologic diagnoses. Understanding the biology underlying skin tone variety and ethnic practices congruent with their associated needs is invaluable to any physician who wishes to practice efficient and expert care, especially to pediatric patients of this category.

Many dermatologic conditions common in the pediatric population may have unique presentations in skin of color or occur with greater incidence in this population. This may be due to ethnic origin, socioeconomic factors, or other influences. Awareness of the potential clinical variations in skin of color may enhance prompt diagnosis, appropriate treatment, and/or reassurance as indicated.

Pediatric dermatology is an incredibly rewarding field. Children are resilient and just want to know that you are advocating for their best interests. Teaming up with children and their parents can lead to fantastic therapeutic alliances and successes. The author has divided this chapter based on a handful of common pediatric dermatologic diseases and what he sees as some of the main clinical and therapeutic tips and tricks that have helped him in his practice.

Language is used to convey thought, but it also influences thought and perception, in turn affecting health care delivery. In this review, we seek to highlight ways in which dermatologists can incorporate inclusive language into practice. By using patient-centered and patient-affirming language, avoiding labels, and naming medical conditions with terminology rooted in pathophysiology rather than outmoded, racist convention or eponyms, dermatologists can strengthen therapeutic relationships and improve patient care.

Pediatric populations are expected to bear most of the climate change impacts, with racial minorities and children living in poorer countries being particularly vulnerable. Given their relevance to cutaneous disease, dermatologists should be aware of these climate-sensitive health impacts and the ways in which they intersect with social factors. Strategies including targeted risk communication, motivational interviewing, and storytelling can help facilitate climate discussions during the patient encounter. In this article the authors summarize common dermatologic health impacts related to environmental exposures and provide sample scripts for climate messaging.

DERMATOLOGIC CLINICS

SERIES OF RELATED INTEREST

Medical Clinics
https://www.medical.theclinics.com/
Immunology and Allergy Clinics
https://www.immunology.theclinics.com/
Clinics in Plastic Surgery
https://www.plasticsurgery.theclinics.com/

THE CLINICS ARE AVAILABLE ONLINE!
Access your subscription at:
www.theclinics.com

Preface

The Science, Art, and Delivery of Pediatric Dermatologic Care in the Twenty-First Century

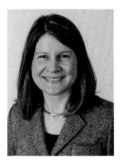

Kelly M. Cordoro, MD
Editor

Caring for children with skin disease is in equal measure rewarding and challenging. Managing patients with diverse backgrounds in the context of complex diagnoses, patient age, developmental stage, and beliefs and preferences of caregivers requires unique knowledge, skills, and strategies. In an era of rapid advancements in diagnosis and treatment, we must also remain cognizant of sociocultural evolution and environmental factors that should factor into our provision of care. Advocating for the vulnerable, providing access, abandoning outdated lexicons, and empowering patients by sharing information and decisions are important aspects of multidimensional care. This issue of *Dermatologic Clinics* features a stellar lineup of authors who take us on a deep dive into challenging issues that arise in daily practice. From clinically relevant genetic testing, an updated approach to epidermal nevi and pigmented lesions, bedside diagnostics, innovative treatments, cultural competence, and communication pearls, each article resonates with the voice of sage teachers and the experience of master clinicians. The authors guide us through clinical quandaries, such as ancillary testing for atypical Spitz nevi, melanonychia, multiple café-au-lait macules, and epidermal nevus syndromes. They arm us with information to navigate common questions and dispel the myths of melanocytic nevi and offer clever treatment pearls for common skin conditions. Normal and pathologic skin findings in pediatric patients with skin of color are skillfully reviewed with an emphasis on awareness of cultural practices that will elevate care and connection with patients. The authors analyze climate change and its influence on skin disease that will inform our clinical approach by presenting compelling information and real-world examples. A thoughtful reappraisal of lexicon and language offers a rich opportunity to consider the effects

Dermatol Clin 40 (2022) ix–x
https://doi.org/10.1016/j.det.2021.09.010
0733-8635/22/© 2021 Published by Elsevier Inc.

of word choice, pronouns, eponyms, and disease designations that may be offensive, inaccurate, nonaffirming, or exclusive. It is a privilege to have worked with and learned from each of the outstanding authors whose work, experience, and expertise are highlighted in this issue. I invite you to immerse yourself in the words on these pages and incorporate the lessons, wisdom, and pearls into your practice. Our patients will be the beneficiaries of the immense efforts and offerings of these generous and dedicated authors. Thank you.

Kelly M. Cordoro, MD
Division of Pediatric Dermatology
UCSF Dermatology
1701 Divisadero Street
San Francisco, CA 94115, USA

E-mail address:
kelly.cordoro@ucsf.edu

Update on Clinically Relevant Genetic Testing in Pediatric Dermatology

Kevin P. Boyd, MD[a], Faizal Z. Asumda, MD[b], Jennifer L. Hand, MD[a,b,c],*

KEYWORDS

- Whole-exome sequencing • Chromosomal microarray • Karyotype • Fbroblast culture
- Ehlers–Danlos

KEY POINTS

- New genetic technology is available for clinical use.
- Testing options include whole-exome sequencing (WES), fibroblast culture, chromosomal microarray, and others.
- Clinical diagnostic criteria guide appropriate genetic testing. Ehlers–Danlos syndrome updates are highlighted.
- The appropriate test is essential for a correct diagnosis. This article reviews testing distinctions important for pediatric dermatologists.

Since the complete sequencing of the human genome in 2003, access to genetic testing continues to grow. A genetic test generally matches the size of error it is aiming to detect. Karyotype, for example, detects derangements large enough to disrupt visible chromosome banding. Chromosomal microarray (CMA), however, is useful when a smaller deletion or duplication including multiple genes is suspected. Molecular tests offer finer tools, useful when a genetic change as small as a single base pair is considered. Here, we review the major types of genetic testing with a focus on technology useful for pediatric dermatologists.

KARYOTYPE

Karyotyping [**Fig. 1**] is a clinically useful genome-wide "big-picture" snapshot of chromosomal structure.[1,2] Because one-third of human genes regulate cognitive function, a chromosome imbalance large enough to be seen by light microscope is generally associated with severe cognitive deficits and major congenital anomalies. When an absent or extra chromosome is suspected, karyotype is a first-tier test. Further, cytogenetic analysis of chromosomal banding in a karyotype enables the detection of genetic changes involving large sections that include at least several megabases (Mb) of DNA.[1,2] Karyotypes can be prepared from a variety of clinical samples including peripheral blood (leukocytes), bone marrow, tumor biopsies, skin biopsy (fibroblasts), amniotic fluid, and chorionic villus for prenatal diagnosis.[1–3] In general, blood is an optimal sample source when chromosomal aneuploidies or structural changes are suspected. Bone marrow biopsy can be used in certain cancers or blood disorders. Soft tissue tumor cells can be used for tumor-specific testing and skin biopsy for fibroblasts is an option in the event of fetal demise. The basic process requires cells that have been arrested during cell division. Karyotype is useful because metaphase chromosomes are captured

[a] Department of Dermatology, Mayo Clinic, 200 1st Street Southwest, Rochester, MN 55905, USA;
[b] Department of Clinical Genomics, Mayo Clinic, 200 1st Street Southwest, Rochester, MN 55905, USA;
[c] Department of Pediatric and Adolescent Medicine, Mayo Clinic, 200 1st Street Southwest, Rochester, MN 55905, USA
* Corresponding author.
E-mail address: hand.jennifer@mayo.edu
Twitter: @jlh8515 (J.L.H.)

Dermatol Clin 40 (2022) 1–8
https://doi.org/10.1016/j.det.2021.08.001
0733-8635/22/© 2021 Elsevier Inc. All rights reserved.

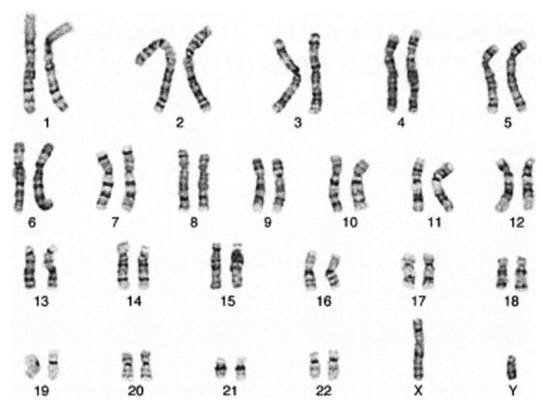

Fig. 1. Karyotyping, Normal human male karyotype, showing 22 pairs of autosomes, one X chromosome, and one Y chromosome. (*From* Chiang VW and Zaoutis LB. Comprehensive Pediatric Hospital Medicine. Elsevier Inc., 2007. *Reproduced with permission* of Chiang VW and Zaoutis LB.)

in their most contracted and recognizable form.[3] Direct view of the chromosomes is not possible in any other type of genetic testing. Chromosomes are stained to generate characteristic banding patterns with structural details of each chromosome observable under a light microscope.[1,2] Analysis of the banding patterns enables the detection of chromosomal changes such as deletions, duplications, translocations, inversions, and low-level mosaicism.[1,2] One practical aspect to be aware of when requesting a karyotype is the resolution which refers to the total number of bands visible in one haploid set of chromosomes. One band equals roughly 6 Mb of DNA. Karyotype resolutions generally range from 400 to 800 bands. High-resolution karyotypes (greater than 550 bands) are more likely to detect smaller structural abnormalities.

Ordering a karyotype in children is often related to the assessment of dysmorphism and clinical features. Classic facial features and cutaneous manifestations may be noted in early life, and if characteristic features of a chromosome disorder are identified or at least suspected, karyotype is the optimal choice for confirming the diagnosis. Only certain numeric chromosome abnormalities are compatible with human life, examples of which include Down (trisomy 21), Edward (trisomy 18), Patau (trisomy 13), Klinefelter (XXY), and Turner (monosomy X) syndromes. Of these, the following are most relevant to pediatric dermatologists. Down syndrome is the most common, and, given its frequency, a dermatologist might pick up on subtle clues in an infant. If a neonate is noted to have multiple major congenital anomalies without features of an obvious syndrome and a numeric chromosome anomaly is suspected, karyotype is again a preferred first-line test. Additionally relevant to pediatric dermatologists is the evaluation of neonatal aplasia cutis which can occur sporadically or associated with additional anomalies. Cutis aplasia in a large stellate pattern may be associated with trisomy 13 (Patau syndrome).

CHROMOSOMAL MICROARRAY

CMA or "molecular karyotyping" has a finer resolution than a traditional karyotype and is increasingly used as a first-tier diagnostic test for a spectrum of disorders including those with multiple congenital anomalies and associated dermatologic pathologies.[4–6] The diagnostic yield for CMA is several orders higher than karyotyping (15%–20% vs

3%) in individuals with unexplained developmental delay, intellectual disability, and multiple congenital anomalies excluding severe more recognizable chromosomal syndromes such as trisomies 13, 18, and 21.[4–6] Primary indications for CMA include primary screening for patients with dysmorphic features, birth defects, intellectual disability, multiple congenital anomalies, and in cases of suspected partial chromosomal imbalance.[4] It is also used to determine chromosomal breakpoints and to distinguish whole-chromosome uniparental disomy in children with imprinting disorders.[4] CMA encompasses different types of array-based genomic copy number variation analyses such as microarray-based comparative genomic hybridization (aCGH) and single-nucleotide polymorphism (SNP) array.[4–6] These techniques enable the visualization of chromosomal rearrangements including gains and losses at a much higher resolution than karyotyping.[4] Whole-genome CMA involves the placement of millions of probes throughout the genome for the detection of copy number variants.[4] DNA deletions ≥ 25 kilobases (kb) and duplications as small as ≥ 50 kb can be identified.[4] The key limitation for CMA is its inability to detect balanced chromosomal rearrangements (inversions, balanced insertions, and balanced translocations) as well as low level mosaicism.[4] Sample preparation for CMA does not require live cells and can include formalin-fixed and paraffin-embedded samples as well as skin biopsies.[4]

This genetic testing method is useful for dermatologists because it can discover small chromosomal aberrations (microdeletions) that would be missed by karyotype given the increased resolution (down to 100 kb) but cannot identify balanced translocations. This method can be used to diagnose microdeletion syndromes such as Prader–Willi and Angelman syndromes. These classic microdeletion syndromes affect the same region of chromosome 15 that includes the gene encoding oculocutaneous albinism type 2 (OCA2). As a result, these patients can have fairer skin, notable as a lighter Fitzpatrick skin type on dermatology exam[7–9] In a child with hypopigmentation along with cognitive deficits and seizures, a chromosomal microdeletion associated with Angelman syndrome should be considered.

Seen almost entirely in males, recessive X-linked ichthyosis (RXLI) is another important microdeletion syndrome. Present in about one out of every 2000 males,[10] RXLI is second only to ichthyosis vulgaris among disorders of keratinization. The STS gene is disrupted by a chromosomal microdeletion in 80% to 90% of cases.[11] When suspected, the diagnosis can be confirmed through CMA, keeping in mind that cases are caused by point mutations will be missed using this method. CMA provides the benefit of detecting not only the presence but also the size of a pathogenic deletion. A typical deletion includes roughly 1.5 Mb of DNA and includes a few genes on one or both sides of the STS gene. A still larger deletion that includes several genes may result in a "contiguous gene syndrome" with characteristic hypogonadotropic hypogonadism and anosmia seen in Kallmann syndrome or epiphyseal stippling seen in X-linked chondrodysplasia punctata.

An evaluation of an infant or young child for a congenital cutaneous concern should include a head-to-toe skin examination to assess for additional anomalies. With the associated developmental delay, intellectual disability, or autism, CMA is the test of choice. A common scenario for pediatric dermatologists relates to congenital anomalies in the form of birthmarks such as epidermal nevi or vascular malformations or to generalized skin changes such as ichthyosis. If a careful evaluation and review of systems reveal development delay or other congenital anomalies and a syndromic diagnosis is not clear, a CMA test is an appropriate place to start. As noted above, CMA is now considered a first-line test in this type of situation. Since about one-third of genes are thought to control brain function, if there is developmental delay without the pattern of major congenital abnormality seen in whole chromosome disorders, it is more likely that a copy number error that includes more than one gene in deletion or duplication is present. This presentation is common in children with autism or developmental delays too subtle to have been noticed as a major disorder at birth. These children may be recognized in dermatology clinic closer to school age in the setting of a congenital skin disorder or birthmark. CMA is considered a first-line test.

SINGLE-GENE DISORDERS

For disorders in which the disruption of a single gene is suspected, targeted testing via single-gene or multi-gene panels is now possible with next-generation sequencing (NGS) technology.[12–14] This category of testing offers a more focused analysis of a certain gene or genes when the clinical evaluation suggests either a specific disorder or a group of disorders that share overlapping features. Genes can now be analyzed with sequencing and deletion duplication technology with turnaround time as fast as 1 or 2 weeks.[12] This technique is highly dependent on the clinical evaluation which guides the specific gene(s) to be tested. A highly focused and complete analysis of clinically relevant genes offers a better chance of diagnosis.

The number of known mutations associated with specific diseases has continued to grow. A better understanding of molecular regulatory pathways has improved the classification of related genes into single panel-type genetic tests for groups of disorders that share overlapping features. Further, the result for a targeted genetic test usually includes information about the diagnosis associated with a particular mutation and also the precise location of the genetic mutation within the gene and the type of mutation. Most testing result reports classify a genetic variant as "pathogenic," "likely pathogenic," "likely benign," or "benign" based on several factors. Prior published reports and predicted protein changes drawn from computer molecular modeling contribute to the decision to classify a mutation as pathogenic or not. In some cases, available data are insufficient to classify a variant and the result will be called a "Variant of Undetermined Significance (VUS)." In genetic testing, a "negative" result does not completely rule out a disease or diagnosis because it is possible a causative genetic change is present, but undetectable based on the limits of current technology. Patients who meet clinical diagnostic criteria are recommended to undergo annual surveillance for their disorder even when molecular testing does not confirm a diagnosis. For example, screening for Wilms tumor is recommended until age 8 years for a child with Megalencephaly-capillary malformation syndrome. Periodic genetics follow-up is recommended, usually every 3 to 4 years, for updated testing and evaluation of any new clinical features in the patient and family that may suggest a different diagnosis.

In the case of a patient who does not meet diagnostic criteria for NF1 and has features that are shared by several RASopathy disorders, a preferred testing strategy may be to choose a test that includes several RASopathy disorders at the outset of the evaluation. Panel-style tests are particularly useful in patients with overlapping phenotypic findings of genetically related disorders. Members of the group of disorders called RASopathies include Neurofibromatosis type I (NF1), cardiofaciocutaneous, Noonan, Noonan with multiple lentigines (previously called LEOPARD), Costello, and Legius syndrome. Although each of these syndromes is caused by a different mutated gene, each affected gene encodes a different member of the same RAS/mitogen-activated protein kinase (MAPK) regulatory pathway. As a result, patients with one of these disorders are likely to have overlapping features such as facial dysmorphia (upside-down triangle-shaped face, outwardly down-slanting palpebral fissures, low-set ears), cognitive deficits, and skin pigmentation changes. Other commonly used multi-gene panel tests include an autoinflammatory panel to evaluate a child with suspected periodic fever or the use of a multi-cancer panel to evaluate a person with a history of more than one melanoma.

A testing strategy for patients who meet diagnostic criteria for NF1 is usually clear. Typically, for these patients, targeted testing for a mutation in *neurofibromin* (the gene altered in NF1) will take place. Laboratories commonly offer a reflex testing strategy to add testing for a mutation in *SPRED1* which causes Legius syndrome (clinically very closely mimics NF1, but is much less common) if no NF1 mutation is found. Therefore, testing for Legius syndrome is only recommended after NF1 testing shows no mutation.

WHOLE-EXOME AND WHOLE-GENOME SEQUENCING

Whole-exome sequencing (WES) and whole-genome sequencing (WGS) are forms of NGS that offer a more comprehensive screen of the human genome, although a less thorough evaluation of each specific gene. WES analyzes only the expressed or protein-coding regions of the human genome, which account for roughly 2% of genetic material, whereas whole-genome screening, if clinically available, is able to interrogate almost all of the genome including the noncoding DNA. In the search for disease-causing mutations, exomes are a preferred target because greater than 85% of disease-causing mutations known to cause human disease have been identified in the protein-coding regions known as exons.[9] WES, in some research samples, has a diagnostic yield of up to 25%[15] and has a higher rate of finding variants of undetermined significance (VUS). Although the VUS may not yield diagnostic information, they can be put aside for future study and reclassification as an understanding of the genome improves. Changes to medical management and the use of reproduction technologies such as preimplantation diagnosis are not recommended by a VUS. In these cases, medical management falls to the clinical assessment of the patient and family history. Since the classification of a VUS is likely to change to either pathogenic or benign over time, periodic follow-up is recommended. Similarly, periodic follow-up and surveillance are recommended for those who meet clinical criteria for a disorder in the face of negative testing.

The authors only order these complex tests with support from a team of genetics professionals. Members are trained to collect and electronically store family history information, provide informed consent, and follow-up on results that require testing of close family members for interpretation. WES is generally not recommended as a first-line test. Other testing according to the clinical features with consideration of karyotype, CMA, and clinically guided single-gene testing is recommended first. Targeted testing for single-gene disorders, unlike WES, includes nonexpressed areas of the genome and is guided by the patient's clinical examination and history. Also, unlike WES, targeted testing for single genes of interest is optimized to identify common mutations, deletions, duplications relevant to the patient phenotype. For example, in a patient with oculocutaneous albinism, targeted testing for relevant mutations is more likely to confirm a diagnosis than WES. WES is also more likely to miss disease-causing mutations outside the expressed DNA in the genes of interest. Until recently, WGS has been considered too expensive and impractical to be clinically useful, but it is beginning to be available in some clinics.

WGS and WES are considered "unbiased" testing methods in that they do not target strictly candidate genes as would be done with gene panels. The consent process for WES/WGS and documentation and ownership of associated computer-generated data is more complex. In some WES testing methods, DNA from 2 family members and the patient are tested at the same time as a "trio." Often both parents of an affected child make up the trio, but the inclusion of another close relative is also an option. Correlation of different genetic variants and clinical features in multiple family members aid in the determination of the pathogenicity and clinical relevance of a VUS. For the pediatric dermatologist, genetics referral for WES testing could be particularly useful if features of more than one major group of disorders overlap in a single complex patient.[9] For example, a child with ichthyosis and periodic episodes of severe, life-threatening pustular psoriasis may be an ideal candidate for WES. Next-generation tests such as WES and WGS are well-suited to cases for which a specialist's experience denotes a patient's clinical features are atypical of previously recognized disorders.

FIBROBLAST CULTURE

Human dermal fibroblasts are mesenchymal-derived cells that are easily obtained from the skin via punch biopsy. Fibroblasts are especially useful for genetic testing and for disease modeling because they maintain the genetic background of the patient in culture. Fibroblasts can be efficiently isolated and cultured from punch biopsy specimens using commercially available cell culture kits with predefined cell culture media. Any skin fragment can be cultured although material from the forearm area is typically used.[16,17] In the laboratory, dermis is dissected away from skin sample and placed in culture. Adherent fibroblast cells are typically seen after 3 to 4 days and will rapidly proliferate over days to be used for downstream genetic analyses.[16–19] The utility of cultured fibroblasts is that all types of genetic testing as reviewed in this article can be performed on fibroblast-derived DNA. Although DNA isolated directly from the skin without culturing can be used for sequencing, skin DNA without fibroblast culture is not suitable for karyotype.[19] Karyotype is the only test that allows the visualization of the chromosome structure so that balanced rearrangements and numeric chromosome abnormalities can be seen directly and requires a culture to for cells to achieve metaphase. Once isolated and cultured, fibroblasts can be indefinitely stored preferably in liquid nitrogen or at −80° C.[16]

Particularly relevant for dermatology practice is a fibroblast's superior ability to retain its genetic make-up in *mosaic disorders*. Blood samples are less useful because mutated lymphocytes tend to drop out of the blood by apoptosis making their mutations undetectable by routing genetic testing. Fibroblast culture from affected skin is the next step when thorough genetic testing of blood test fails to confirm a clinically suspected diagnosis because the disorder is present in a mosaic form. On the other hand, some disorders such as Proteus and McCune–Albright syndromes are always present in a mosaic state; testing affected tissue is more likely to confirm the diagnosis and is recommended as first-line (rather than blood).[20,21] So-called "Blaschkoid dyspigmentation" is considered a marker for genetic mosaicism. In cases associated with skin as well as major extracutaneous anomalies, karyotype from skin fibroblasts provides a method to confirm a genetic cause if blood testing fails. A recent study of 73 patients with pigmentary mosaicism and extracutaneous anomalies revealed that 9 patients were found to have genetic abnormalities detected by fibroblast culture of both light and dark colored skin areas, but normal karyotype from peripheral blood.[22]

Skin fibroblasts also have importance in gene therapy. In recent decades, induced pluripotent stem cell (iPSC) reprogramming has broadened the clinical utility of fibroblasts as a system for disease modeling.[16,17] Fibroblasts are now routinely reprogrammed into iPSCs via ectopic expression of reprograming factors.[23,24] In essence, a patient's fibroblasts can be reprogrammed to produce patient-specific cells that are amenable to differentiation into various cell types. Fibroblast-derived iPSCs have been differentiated into relevant skin cells including keratinocytes, melanocytes, and demonstrated to form epidermis and skin appendages.[25] This system provides an excellent opportunity for dermatology—some of the most severe forms of inherited skin disease are often caused by known monogenic defects which can in theory be corrected.[26,27] For example, patient-derived fibroblasts can be reprogrammed into pluripotent stem cells, followed by the correction of the specific monogenic defect, and differentiation into autologous skin cells for transplantation.[26,27] At the research level, patient-derived iPSCs are being used for in vitro disease modeling and in vivo xenograft modeling[27,28] to further our understanding of mechanisms of disease pathophysiology and for drug discovery. iPSCs have been derived for a variety of dermatologic pathologies including type VII collagen deficit recessive dystrophic epidermolysis bullosa (RDEB).[28]

BENCH TO BEDSIDE: UPDATED EHLERS–DANLOS DIAGNOSTIC CRITERIA

Clinical diagnostic criteria for various diseases guide genetic testing. It is worth mentioning that diagnostic criteria for Ehlers–Danlos syndrome (EDS) were significantly updated in 2017. The 6 primary types continue to be linked to mutations within collagen-encoding genes, and additional subtypes have been described and linked to unique mutations.[29] Although superb diagnostic genetic testing is available for some forms of EDS, a causative mutation has still not been found for the most common hypermobile type. Since genetic testing is not likely to confirm a diagnosis, clinical delineation of the hypermobile type is useful in deciding whether to perform testing in a particular patient. The Ehlers–Danlos Society has created a checklist to assist physicians of all disciplines in making the diagnosis of the hypermobile type of EDS and this spectrum. The link is provided later in discussion.

- Diagnostic Criteria for Hypermobile Ehlers–Danlos syndrome (hEDS) https://www.ehlers-danlos.com/heds-diagnostic-checklist/

RESOURCES

As the landscape of genetic testing becomes more broad and complex, collaborating with genetics experts is critical, when available. The American College of Medical Genetics maintains a link on their web site titled "Find A Genetic Service;" for clinicians who may not have a Genomics Department available: https://clinics.acmg.net/

SUMMARY

Although the utility of molecular genetic testing has rocketed forward, karyotyping remains a useful tool particularly in the diagnosis of suspected chromosomal disorders. In disorders severe enough to suspect multiple genes are altered, CMA testing is the best first step. For suspected single-gene disorders, targeted single and multigene panels are an increasingly useful means of making a diagnosis. Panel type tests containing multiple specific genes are especially useful in patients with overlapping features of multiple disorders. The number of approved clinical, commercially available tests continues to increase as costs continue to decrease. Due to improved technology and efficient, automated laboratory machines, WES/WGS has become attainable as a send-out test in many clinics. Although not suitable as first-line testing in most circumstances, they may be of particular benefit when other methods do not reveal a diagnosis. Human skin fibroblast culture has special utility for genetic testing in dermatology. Skin fibroblasts are an easily accessible cell source for genetic material that can be indefinitely stored and used for all forms of genetic testing. Skin fibroblasts are superior for the diagnosis of mosaic disorders. Finally, the ability to evaluate patients using clinical diagnostic criteria is essential to guide correct genetic testing. Recent major updates in the diagnostic criteria for Ehlers–Danlos syndrome, for example, aim to make phenotype-based genetic testing more efficient and accurate.

CLINICS CARE POINTS

- Karyotype provides the best "big-picture" view of the genome.
- Karyotype is preferred for suspected major chromosome anomalies such as trisomy 13 or trisomy 21.

- In neonates, large, stellate aplasia cutis is suspicious for trisomy 13 when presenting with other major congenital anomalies.
- CMA has a finer resolution than karyotype; chromosomal copy number errors (deletions and duplications) are large enough to include several genes but too small to be seen by karyotype are best detected using this method.
- In children with multiple minor congenital anomalies (eg, epidermal nevi) and developmental delay, CMA is an appropriate first test.
- For X-linked ichthyosis (RXLI), CMA detects cases (80%–90%) caused by a microdeletion.
- CMA is the best to detect "contiguous gene syndromes" such as Kallmann syndrome or X-linked chondrodysplasia punctata
- For suspected single-gene disorders, targeted testing offers focused, more complete analysis of certain relevant genes when the clinical evaluation suggests a specific disorder or a group of disorders.
- Panel type tests that include several genes are useful for disorders that share overlapping clinical features.
- WES is useful when more targeted testing does not provide a diagnosis.
- WGS is increasingly becoming available for clinical use.
- Human skin fibroblasts provide a superior method to detect mosaic genetic disorders than peripheral blood.
- Knowledge of clinical diagnostic criteria is essential to guide appropriate genetic testing.
- Ehlers–Danlos hypermobility syndrome diagnostic criteria have been updated and are available in a convenient check box format at the Ehlers–Danlos Society website: https://www.ehlers-danlos.com/heds-diagnostic-checklist/

DISCLOSURE

J.L. Hand is a section editor for genetic skin disorders at UpToDate, Inc. The authors have no other disclosures.

REFERENCES

1. Gartler SM. The chromosome number in humans: a brief history. Nat Rev Genet 2006;7:655–60.
2. Speicher MR, Ballard SG, Ward DC. Karyotyping human chromosomes by combinatorial multi-fluor FISH. Nat Genet 1996;12:368–75.
3. Caspersson T, Zech L, Johansson J. Differential banding of alkylating fluorochromes in human chromosomes. Exp Cell Res 1970;60:315–9.
4. Miller DT, Adam MP, Aradhya S, et al. Consensus statement: chromosomal microarray is a first-tier clinical diagnostic test for individuals with developmental disabilities or congenital anomalies. Am J Hum Genet 2010;86:749–64.
5. Nelson R. Whole exome sequencing and chromosomal microarray analysis feasible and cost effective in underserved population. Am J Med Genet 2018;176(5):1044–5.
6. Clark MM, Stark Z, Farnaes L, et al. Meta-analysis of the diagnostic and clinical utility of genome and exome sequencing and chromosomal microarray in children with suspected genetic diseases. NPJ Genom Med 2018;3:16.
7. Lee ST, Nicholls RD, Bundey S, et al. Mutations of the P gene in oculocutaneous albinism, ocular albinism, and Prader-Willi syndrome plus albinism. N Engl J Med 1994;330(8):529–34.
8. Ballabio A, Parent G, Carrozzo R, et al. Isolation and characterization of a steroid sulfatase cDNA clone: genomic deletions in patients with X-chromosome-linked ichthyosis. Proc Natl Acad Sci U S A 1987; 84:4519–23.
9. Chiu FP, Doolan BJ, McGrath JA, et al. A decade of next-generation sequencing in genodermatoses: the impact on gene discovery and clinical diagnostics [published online ahead of print, 2020 Jul 6]. Br J Dermatol 2020. https://doi.org/10.1111/bjd.19384.
10. Brcic L, Underwood JFG, Kendall KM, et al. Medical and neurobehavioral phenotypes in carriers of X-linked ichthyosis-associated genetic deletions in the UK Biobank. J Med Genet 2020;57(10): 692–8.
11. Fernandes NF, Janniger CK, Schwartz RA. X-linked ichthyosis: an oculocutaneous genodermatosis. J Am Acad Dermatol 2010;62(3):480–5.
12. Hall MJ, Forman AD, Pilarski R, et al. Gene panel testing for inherited cancer risk. J Natl Compr Canc Netw 2014;12(9):1339–46.
13. Rizzo JM, Buck MJ. Key principles and clinical applications of "next-generation" DNA sequencing. Cancer Prev Res (Phila) 2012;5:887–900.
14. Linnarsson S. Recent advances in DNA sequencing methods: general principles of sample preparation. Exp Cell Res 2010;316:1339–43.
15. Yang Y, Muzny DM, Reid JG, et al. Clinical whole-exome sequencing for the diagnosis of mendelian disorders. N Engl J Med 2013;369(16):1502–11.
16. Kisiel MA, Klar AS. Isolation and culture of human dermal fibroblasts. Methods Mol Biol 2019;1993: 71–8.
17. Lynch MD, Watt FM. Fibroblast heterogeneity: implications for human disease. J Clin Invest 2018; 128(1):26–35.

18. Stanyon R, Galleni L. A rapid fibroblast culture technique for high resolution karyotypes. Ital J Zoolog 1991;58(1):81–3.

19. Allahbakhshian-Farsani M, Abdian N, Ghasemi-Dehkordi P, et al. Cytogentic analysis of human dermal fibroblasts (HDFs) in early and late passages using both karyotyping and comet assay techniques. Cytotechnology 2014;66(5):815–22.

20. Biesecker LG, Sapp JC. In: Adam MP, Ardinger HH, Pagon RA, et al, editors. GeneReviews® [Internet]. Seattle (WA): University of Washington, Seattle; 1993-2021; 2012. Available at: https://www.ncbi.nlm.nih.gov/books/NBK99495/.

21. Boyce AM, Florenzano P, de Castro LF, et al. Fibrous dysplasia/mccune-albright syndrome. In: Adam MP, Ardinger HH, Pagon RA, et al, editors. GeneReviews® [Internet]. Seattle (WA): University of Washington, Seattle; 1993-2021; 2015. Available at: https://www.ncbi.nlm.nih.gov/books/NBK274564/.

22. Salas-Labadía C, Gómez-Carmona S, Cruz-Alcívar R, et al. Genetic and clinical characterization of 73 Pigmentary Mosaicism patients: revealing the genetic basis of clinical manifestations. Orphanet J Rare Dis 2019;14:259.

23. Takahashi K, Tanabe K, Ohnuki M, et al. Induction of pluripotent stem cells from adult human fibroblasts by defined factors. Cell 2007;131:861–72.

24. Aasen T, Raya A, Barrero MJ, et al. Efficient and rapid generation of induced pluripotent stem cells from human keratinocytes. Nat Biotechnol 2008;26: 1276–84.

25. Itoh M, Kiuru M, Cairo MS, et al. Generation of keratinocytes from normal and recessive dystrophic epidermolysis bullosa-induced pluripotent stem cells. Proc Natl Acad Sci U S A 2011;108:8797–802.

26. Ohyama M, Okano H. Promise of human induced pluripotent stem cells in skin regeneration and investigation. J Invest Dermatol 2014;134(3):605–9.

27. Bilousova G, Chen J, Roop DR. Exploring the therapeutic potential of induced pluripotent stem cells for the treatment of epidermolytic hyperkeratosis and epidermolysis bullosa simplex. J Invest Dermatol 2011;131:S70 (abstract).

28. Bilousova G, Chen J, Roop DR. Differentiation of mouse induced pluripotent stem cells into a multipotent keratinocyte lineage. J Invest Dermatol 2011; 131:857–64.

29. Malfait F, Francomano C, Byers P, et al. The 2017 international classification of the Ehlers-Danlos syndromes. Am J Med Genet C Semin Med Genet 2017;175(1):8–26.

Updated Approach to Patients with Multiple Café au Lait Macules

Mohammed Albaghdadi, MPA[a], My Linh Thibodeau, MD, MSc[b],
Irene Lara-Corrales, MD, MSc[c],*

KEYWORDS

- Cafe au lait macules • CALMs • NF1 • Legius • SPRED1 • Hyperpigmentation
- Neurocutaneous disorders • Genodermatoses

KEY POINTS

- The differential for café au lait macules is broad and considerations should be made based on the number, size, shape, and distribution of the macules.
- Genetic testing can be helpful in diagnosing neurocutaneous disorders in select patients with multiple café au lait macules, particularly in younger children or in those with atypical clinical presentations.
- Diagnosis and management of conditions associated with café au lait macules are best done using a multidisciplinary team.

BACKGROUND

Café au lait macules (CALMs) are discrete, well-circumscribed, round or oval uniformly pigmented skin macules or patches (**Fig. 1**). The pigmentation of CALMs results from increased melanin content, without melanocytic proliferation, in melanocytes and basal keratinocytes. Despite their name, their pigmentation varies from light to dark brown depending on the person's Fitzpatrick skin type. Their border can be smooth, often described as the "coast of California," or jagged like the "coast of Maine." An atypical CALM is one that has an irregular or smudgy border and nonhomogeneous pigmentation[1–3] (**Fig. 2**). In certain instances like in Fanconi anemia, they present as subtly darker than the surrounding skin with ill-defined edges termed "shadow spots."[4]

In newborns, the size of CALMs ranges from 2 to 40 mm in length and 2 to 35 mm in width and increases proportionally with body growth.[5] In older children and adults, the diameter can range from 15 to 300 mm.[6] The most common locations of CALMs in the newborn and older children are the buttock and trunk, respectively,[5,7] but they can appear anywhere on the body. The location of CALMs suggests that sunlight exposure is not involved in the pathogenesis.[1] There has been no established relationship to melanoma, and CALMs show no tendency toward malignancy.[8]

CAFÉ AU LAIT MACULES DIFFERENTIAL DIAGNOSIS

Although CALMs are easy to diagnose on clinical examination, other pigmented lesions are often mistaken for CALMs. The differential diagnosis includes both congenital and acquired lesions. Congenital melanocytic nevi, speckled lentiginous nevus, and pigmentary mosaicism can be confused with CALMs.[1] Some congenital melanocytic nevi can be light patches at birth and develop

[a] Temerty Faculty of Medicine, University of Toronto, Toronto, Canada; [b] Division of Clinical and Metabolic Genetics, Hospital for Sick Children, University of Toronto, Toronto, Canada; [c] Pediatric Dermatology, Division of Dermatology, Hospital for Sick Children, University of Toronto, 555 University Avenue, Toronto, Ontario M5G1X8, Canada
* Corresponding author.
E-mail address: Irene.lara-corrales@sickkids.ca

derm.theclinics.com

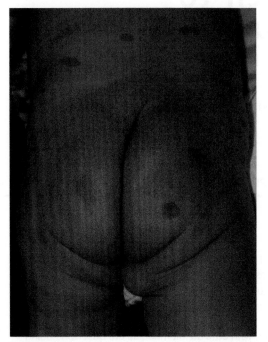

Fig. 1. Typical CALMs present as well demarcated, hyperpigmented macules or patches with uniform pigmentation.

texture and darker pigmentation with time. Pigmentary mosaicism refers to an area of the skin that has a different skin tone when compared with the rest of the skin, and sometimes it might be difficult to tell apart from a large CALM. Acquired lesions that can resemble CALMs include freckles (ephelides), lentigos, and postinflammatory hyperpigmentation. Other mimickers include urticaria pigmentosa and solitary mastocytomas.[1]

INCIDENCE IN THE GENERAL POPULATION

The incidence of CALMs varies depending on the population being studied with estimates between 0.3% and 36% with equal distribution in both sexes.[7,9] Solitary CALMs are common in the general population with most studies reporting between 1 and 3 CALMs.[7,9] In contrast, having multiple CALMs is unusual and may indicate underlying genetic disease. The probability of having 6 or more CALMs in an individual with no underlying genetic disease is less than 0.1%.[10] Specifically, the presence of 6 or more CALMs measuring more than 5 mm in prepubertal individuals, or more than 15 mm in postpubertal individuals, is a clinical criterion for the diagnosis of neurofibromatosis type 1 (NF1).[11] NF1 is the most common condition associated with multiple CALMs, but not the only one.

NEUROFIBROMATOSIS TYPE 1

NF1 is an autosomal dominant systemic disorder with complete penetrance and variable expressivity affecting approximately 1:2000 to 1:4000 individuals.[12,13] About 50% of affected individuals present without a family history, and the condition is de novo.[8,14] A clinical diagnosis is based on the presence of 2 or more features out of 7 criteria outlined in the National Institutes of Health (NIH) consensus statement.[15,16] These criteria were

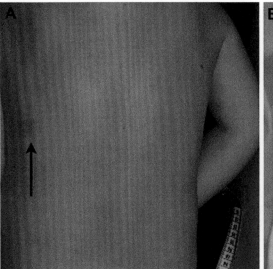
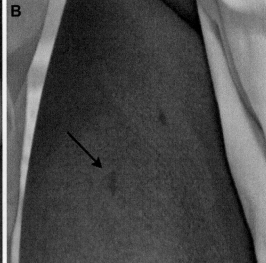

Fig. 2. Atypical CALMs are ill-defined and do not have distinct, well-demarcated borders. Arrows in panels A and B show atypical CALMS.

Table 1
The previous and recently updated National Institutes of Health diagnostic criteria for neurofibromatosis type 1

Cardinal Clinical Features (Any Two or More Are Required for Diagnosis)[15]	New Changes[23]
1. Six or more café-au-lait macules more than 5 mm in greatest diameter in prepubertal individuals and more than 15 mm in greatest diameter in postpubertal individuals	Must be bilateral (both sides of the body)[a]
2. Freckling in the axillary or inguinal regions	Must be bilateral (both sides of the body)[a]
3. Two or more neurofibromas of any type or one plexiform neurofibroma	No change
4. Two or more Lisch nodules	Or 2 or more choroidal abnormalities
5. Optic pathway glioma	No change
6. A distinctive osseous lesion such as sphenoid wing dysplasia	Added anterolateral bowing of tibia (tibial dysplasia), or pseudarthrosis of a long bone
7. First-degree relative (eg, mother, father, sister, brother) with NF1	Changed to a parent with NF1 by the aforementioned criteria
8.	New criteria: A pathogenic NF1 variant

Abbreviation: NIH, National Institutes of Health.
^a If only café au lait macules and freckling are present, the diagnosis is most likely NF1, but exceptionally the person might have another diagnosis such as Legius syndrome. At least 1 of the 2 pigmentary findings (café au lait macules or freckling) should be bilateral.

published in 1988, and there have been recent efforts to update them. See **Table 1** for the current and proposed changes to the criteria.

NF1 shows age-dependent clinical expression. At least 6 or more CALMs are most often the first identifiable feature and are present in all patients with NF1 by 1 year of life.[17] As such, the presence of multiple CALMs is an important red flag to suspect NF1. For patients with NF1, CALMs increase in number and size over time. To be counted for the diagnostic criteria, these should be at least 5 mm in diameter in prepubertal individuals and 15 mm in postpubertal patients.[18]

If only CALMs are present, a clinical diagnosis of NF1 can only be made when a second feature outlined in the NIH criteria develops. This fact is of particular importance for sporadic NF1 cases because there might be a delay in establishing a clinical diagnosis. DeBella and colleagues[17] (2000) estimated that 46% of sporadic NF1 cases will lack 2 or more diagnostic features by 1 year of age. Furthermore, 30% of patients with NF1 younger than 1 year present with only 1 feature, which is typically CALMs.[17] Other features such as plexiform neurofibromas and tibial dysplasia maybe be present within the first year of life, but optic pathway gliomas and axillary freckling may not present until ages 3 to 7 years[18,19] (**Fig. 3**).

SIX OR MORE CAFÉ AU LAIT MACULES AND NEUROFIBROMATOSIS TYPE 1

Korf[20] (1992) studied children ranging in age from 1 month to 14 years who presented with 6 or

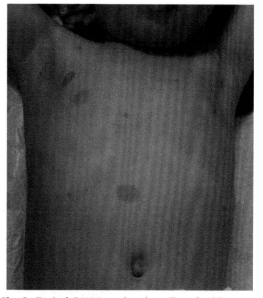

Fig. 3. Typical CALMs and early axillary freckling in a patient with NF1.

more CALMs and no other NF1 features longitudinally over a 9-year period. The results showed that 24 of 41 (59%) went on to develop other features of NF1. Furthermore, among those diagnosed with NF1, 75% had a clinical diagnosis before the age of 6 years, and all but 2 had a diagnosis before the age of 10 years. Finally, the investigator notes that 8 of 41 (20%) patients who did not develop NF1 were younger than the rest of the cohort, which could suggest that they could go on to develop other signs of NF1 with time. This observation highlights the importance of clinical suspicion of NF1 in patients with multiple CALMs and the need for follow-up.

Nunley and colleagues[2] (2009) found that 77% of children who had 6 or more typical CALMs at the initial presentation were eventually diagnosed with NF1, and of those diagnosed with NF1, all of them met the NIH criteria by age 8 years. Those who were eventually diagnosed with NF1 had a higher mean number of CALMs at their initial presentation (11.8 CALMs) when compared with those who did not (4.6 CALMs). Furthermore, all those diagnosed with NF1 had more than 6 CALMs. Importantly, the shape of the CALMs mattered diagnostically, because only 5% of those with atypical CALMs were diagnosed with NF1. As such, the morphologic characteristics of the CALMs offer diagnostic value.

In a more recent study, Ben-Shachar et al.[3] (2017) developed an algorithm to detect the risk of having constitutional NF1 based on the number and shape of isolated CALMs without other stigmata of NF1 using a clinical and molecular cohort. The investigators stratified their patients into 3 risk groups: high risk, intermediate risk, and low risk of having NF1.

- The high-risk group: These patients had 6 or more CALMs and were younger than 29 months. Patients with 6 or more CALMs and younger than 14 months were considered to be very high risk. Overall, the high-risk group had an 80.4% chance of developing NF1.
- The intermediate-risk group: These patients had less than 6 CALMs and were younger than 29 months, or they had 6 or more CALMs and were older than 29 months without atypical CALMs. The intermediate-risk group had between 11.5% and 14.3% chance of developing NF1.
- The low-risk group: These patients had less than 6 CALMs and were older than 29 months or were older than 29 months and had atypical CALMs. The low-risk group had a 0.9% chance of developing constitutional NF1.

The investigators tried simplifying the age cutoffs to 12, 30, and 72 months (1, 2.5, and 6 years, respectively) and that had a similar predictive result. The results from this article could help identify patients who would benefit from early genetic testing to confirm a diagnosis of NF1 based on their risk. Specifically, those in the high-risk group that have 6 more CALMs and are younger than 2.5 years have a high pretest probability of having a pathogenic variant on genetic testing.

GENETIC TESTING FOR NEUROFIBROMATOSIS TYPE 1

Comprehensive RNA-based genetic testing for NF1 using lymphocytes has a sensitivity of 95%.[21] Some genotype-phenotype correlations have recently emerged. For example, a base pair in-frame deletion in exon 17 of the NF1 gene resulted in a clinical phenotype with no cutaneous neurofibromas or plexiform neurofibromas.[22] However, the NF1 gene is large, making genotype-phenotype correlations challenging. In most cases, genetic testing can confirm clinical suspicion for NF1 and is essential for ongoing surveillance, management, and reproductive counseling; thus genetic testing for molecular diagnostic confirmation is favored by experts and has been added as a new clinical criterion in the updated NIH diagnostic criteria (see **Table 1**).[23] However, completing genetic testing in all patients presenting with CALMs might not be feasible or accessible. Furthermore, a patient can meet the clinical criteria for NF1, but have negative NF1 gene testing (no molecular disease-causing variant identified). A negative genetic test result does not definitively rule out NF1 because the test is not 100% sensitive and some mutations are not yet discovered or detectable by conventional DNA testing.[21,24] Two key alternative diagnostic possibilities could explain a negative NF1 genetic test result: mosaic neurofibromatosis type 1 (MNF) and Legius syndrome. A few less common diagnoses can be considered as well and will be discussed later in the article.

MOSAIC NEUROFIBROMATOSIS TYPE 1

Patients with MNF can present with features of NF1 like CALMs or freckling in a localized or generalized area of the body, but do not typically have an NF1 germline mutation (**Fig. 4**). The diagnostic criteria have been recently elucidated for MNF and are diagnostic if any of the following is present[23]:

- A pathogenic heterozygous NF1 variant with a variant allele fraction of significantly less than

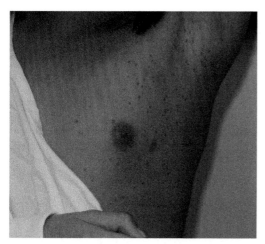

Fig. 4. Unilateral CALMs and axillary freckling in a patient with MNF.

50% in apparently normal tissue such as white blood cells AND one other NF1 diagnostic criterion (except a parent fulfilling the diagnostic criteria for NF1)
- An identical pathogenic heterozygous NF1 variant in 2 anatomically independent affected tissues (in the absence of a pathogenic NF1 variant in unaffected tissue)
- A clearly segmental distribution of café au lait macules or cutaneous neurofibromas AND either another NF1 criteria (except a parent) or a child fulfilling the diagnostic criteria for NF1
- An individual fulfilling only 1 NF1 diagnostic criterion from the following list: freckling in the axillary and inguinal region, optic pathway glioma, 2 or more Lisch nodules or 2 or more choroidal abnormalities, distinctive osseous lesion typical for NF1, 2 or more neurofibromas or 1 plexiform neurofibroma, AND conceived an offspring that fulfills the criteria for NF1

This phenotype is the result of a postzygotic variant that affects only certain tissues (somatic mosaicism), and the specific pattern depends on the timing of the variant and the cell lines involved.[25,26] In the study by Korf[20] (1992) discussed earlier, 15% of the cohort with 6 or more CALMs had a final diagnosis of MNF. The estimated population prevalence of MNF is between 1:36,000 and 1:40,000, which is almost 10 times less frequent than the prevalence of NF1.[25,27] Clinically patients with MNF have a milder phenotype, with less complications associated with NF1, which suggests that the real incidence is likely higher.[28,29] However, MNF should not be minimized because malignancy is still found in up to

13% of reported cases[28,29] and other changes associated with NF1 can present in affected tissues. Furthermore, there have been reported cases of gonadal mosaicism, which has led to constitutional transmission and conventional NF1 in the offspring of individuals with MNF.[30]

Variant testing for MNF through blood lymphocytes is often negative because of low mosaicism levels. In this situation, a tissue diagnosis can be obtained through *NF1* genetic testing on cultured melanocytes obtained from skin biopsies of CALMs. Establishing the diagnosis allows proper surveillance and genetic counseling for affected individuals.

LEGIUS SYNDROME

The primary differential diagnosis for NF1 is Legius syndrome, a genetic disorder that can also present with 6 or more CALMs, axillary freckling, neurocognitive impairment, developmental delay, and macrocephaly. The primary difference from NF1 is the lack of tumors including neurofibromas, optic gliomas, and Lisch nodules and lack of osseous lesions.[31,32] The genetic variants associated with Legius syndrome cause a loss of function in the sprouty-related EVH1 domain-containing protein 1 encoded by the *SPRED1* gene. Based on the NIH criteria, patients with Legius syndrome can meet up to 3 of the diagnostic criteria for NF1. Messiaen and colleagues[31] (2009) showed that half of the patients who tested positive for a *SPRED1* disease-causing variant met the NIH diagnostic criteria for NF1 based on the presence of 6 or more CALMs, axillary/inguinal freckling, and/or a clinically diagnosed NF1 family history. Patients who presented with an NF1-compatible family history and CALMs with or without freckling and no other features tested positive for a pathogenic *SPRED1* variant 19% of the time and for a pathogenic *NF1* variant 73% of the time.[31] The investigators estimated that 1% to 4% of individuals with multiple CALMs harbor a heterozygous *SPRED1* variant and that 2% of those who meet the NF1 clinical criteria from the NIH do not have NF1 but instead have a *SPRED1* variant associated with Legius syndrome.[31]

The distinction between NF1 and Legius syndrome is an important one to make because Legius syndrome is a genetic condition primarily affecting skin pigmentation and is not associated with tumors. However, the pigmentary manifestations that raise suspicion for NF1 overlap significantly, so in the absence of other features like neurofibromas, it is not possible to tell them apart clinically (**Fig. 5**). One research group

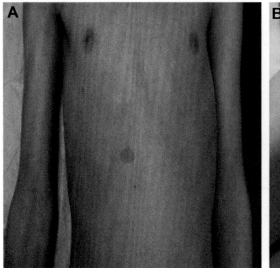 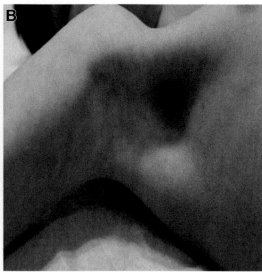

Fig. 5. CALMs (*A*) and axillary freckling (*B*) in a patient with Legius syndrome.

hypothesized that individuals with Legius syndrome may be at increased risk of leukemia based on one patient with a germline *SPRED1* disease-causing variant who developed acute myeloid leukemia, but this association has not been independently validated to date.[33]

Genetic testing can be the only way to distinguish between NF1 and Legius syndrome in some patient populations, particularly in the first few years of life. Many laboratories test for *SPRED1* and *NF1* genes simultaneously, whereas others test *SPRED1* only when *NF1* genetic testing is negative. *SPRED1* gene should be investigated in all cases of suspected NF1 with negative *NF1* genetic testing because a diagnosis of Legius syndrome does not require as rigorous surveillance as NF1.

CAFÉ AU LAIT MACULES AND OTHER GENETIC DISORDERS

CALMs are also associated with several rarer genetic conditions. NF1 is secondary to variants in the *neurofibromin* gene, which is involved in RAS signaling. CALMs have also been identified in other RASopathies such as Noonan syndrome,[34] Noonan syndrome with lentigines,[35] Costello syndrome,[36] and cardiofaciocutaneous syndrome.[37] Genetic syndromes caused by gene variants in the *KITLG/KIT* signaling pathway can also cause CALMs,[38] including piebaldisim[39] and familial progressive hyperpigmentation.[40,41] Other genetic disorders associated with CALMs include Fanconi anemia,[4] ring chromosome syndrome,[42] constitutional mismatch repair deficiency syndrome,[43]

ataxia telangiectasia,[44] and neurofibromatosis type 2.[45]

Neurofibromatosis type 2 (NF2) is an autosomal dominant disorder that results from mutations on chromosome 22. Despite the name, NF2 is a distinct entity from NF1 with little phenotypic overlap. NF2 is clinically characterized by neurologic lesions (bilateral vestibular schwannomas most commonly, intracranial meningiomas, and spinal tumors), ophthalmologic lesions (cataracts), and cutaneous lesions (tumors, plaques). Most cutaneous tumors tend to be schwannomas, although neurofibromas are possible. The plaques are well-circumscribed, slightly raised roughened areas, smaller than 2 cm, pigmented, and with excess hair.[45,46] Although CALMs have been reported in 33% to 48% of patients with this disorder, they are mostly singular and very rarely more than 5.[45,46] Furthermore, they are smaller than the CALMs seen in NF1, are paler, and have more irregular borders.[47]

McCune-Albright syndrome (MAS) is a rare disorder that occurs as a result of a somatic gain-of-function mutation that leads to a mosaic activation of Gα. MAS is described as a triad of CALMs, endocrinopathies, and fibrous dysplasia.[48] CALMs are one of the earliest presenting features of MAS. CALMs in MAS differ from those in NF1 in that they tend to follow the lines of Blaschko (characteristic distribution reminiscent of embryonic cell migration patterns),[49] they respect the midline of the body, their borders tend to be jagged resembling the "Coast of Maine," and they are fewer in number (less than 6), larger in diameter, and darker in pigmentation.[50]

Tuberous sclerosis complex (TSC) is a multisystem disorder caused by mutations in the tumor suppressor gene TSC1 (encoding hamartin) or TSC2 (encoding tuberin) leading to subsequent growth of hamartomas in the brain, kidney, lung, heart, and skin. The cutaneous manifestations are an important aspect in the diagnostic process of TSC. Cutaneous features include facial angiofibromas, hypomelanotic macules (ash leaf, thumbprintlike macules, and confettilike skin lesions), shagreen patches, and periungual or subungual fibromas (Koenen tumors).[51] Although CALMs have been reported with TSC, they are often solitary and are not considered part of the diagnostic criteria for TSC.[52]

There are reports of families presenting with multiple CALMs without any other stigmata of NF1 and no evidence of mutation in the NF1 gene. This condition has been termed multiple café au lait spots (OMIM 613113) and seems to be transmitted in an autosomal dominant fashion.[53–55] Further studies are warranted to determine the genetic underpinnings of this group.

The differentiation between these conditions can be difficult because there exists significant overlap in clinical presentation and genetic testing may be necessary to reach the correct diagnosis. We summarize these genetic conditions associated with CALMs in **Table 2**.

APPROACH TO CAFÉ AU LAIT MACULES

A stepwise approach is helpful early on. The first step is evaluating whether prepubertal patients, especially young children in the first few years of life, present with 6 or more CALMs measuring more than 5 mm, because this would increase our clinical suspicion for NF1. In older patients, if they present with CALMs only, with no other clinical features of NF1 the clinical suspicion is lower.[2,3,17,20] We summarized our approach to multiple typical CALMs in **Figs. 6** and **7**.

CAFÉ AU LAIT MACULES MEETING THE NEUROFIBROMATOSIS TYPE 1 NATIONAL INSTITUTES OF HEALTH CRITERIA

For children with CALMs meeting the NIH criteria, the age of the child is an important consideration. A genetic test for NF1/SPRED1 may be appropriate in very young children (younger than 2.5 years) only meeting the CALMs NIH criteria for NF1. A recent study showed that 21% of patients fulfilling solely the CALMs NIH criteria for NF1 tested positive through genetic testing. The study investigators noted that the NIH criteria may not be sensitive to diagnose NF1 in young

patients and that genetic testing might help.[56] Alternatively, clinical follow-up in 6 to 12 months may be appropriate because children could go on to develop other symptoms and most patients with NF1 will meet the NIH clinical diagnostic criteria by age 8 years.[20] For older children meeting solely the CALMs' NIH criteria for NF1, genetic testing can be offered. Furthermore, depending on the level of clinical suspicion, follow-up yearly can also be considered. For patient with confirmed NF1, following health surveillance guidelines published by the American Academy of Pediatrics is recommended.[12]

In children who meet the CALMs NIH criteria for NF1 and have a parent with confirmed NF1, a clinical diagnosis of NF1 can be made without molecular confirmation. However, Legius syndrome remains a possibility in both the parent and the child if NF1 was diagnosed clinically in the parent and was never genetically confirmed, as was highlighted by Messiaen and colleagues (2009).[31]

In children who present with CALMs and axillary/inguinal freckling without other NIH criteria, we recommend genetic testing to help differentiate between NF1 and Legius syndrome. However, if the child presents with NF1-related tumors as well as other cutaneous manifestations, NF1 should be strongly suspected. MNF can also be considered in this scenario, particularly if genetic testing is negative for NF1 and Legius syndrome.

Clinical suspicion for MNF needs to be high in patients with localized or pattern-based CALMs even when they meet the NF1 CALMs NIH criteria. If *NF1* genetic testing in blood reveals a negative result, even in patients with bilateral skin findings, one should consider MNF. For such patients, genetic testing in tissue can be offered later in their life to confirm a molecular diagnosis and to offer genetic counseling. Confirming the mosaic state early in life will not change management, and because this is an invasive procedure, it might be best to wait until the patient can understand and consent for the testing. Counseling regarding family planning and possible gonadal mosaicism can also be offered later in life, once a molecular diagnosis is confirmed. There are no specific health surveillance guidelines for patients with confirmed or suspected MNF. Because patients with MNF have a milder phenotype, less frequent health monitoring is often suggested.

For children who meet the NIH clinical criteria, but test negative for NF1/SPRED1 or test positive for a variant of unknown significance (VUS) for NF1/SPRED1, we recommend clinical follow-up as if they have NF1 and monitoring for NF1-related complications. The genetic test for NF1/SPRED1 can be repeated if more sensitive testing

Table 2
Conditions featuring café au lait macules

Condition	Gene (Inheritance)	Associated Features[a]	Additional Testing to Consider
Ataxia telangiectasia	ATM (AR)	Progeric changes in skin and hair, hypopigmented macules, progressive neurologic impairment, cerebellar ataxia, radiosensitivity, malignancy, immunocompromise, premature aging, and oculocutaneous telangiectasia	Karyotype[a] Serum AFP[a]
Cardio faciocutaneous syndrome	BRAF, MAP2K1/2 (AD)	Follicular hyperkeratosis, sparse slow-growing curly hair, ulerythema ophryogenes, melanocytic nevi, infantile hemangiomas, distinctive craniofacial features, cardiac anomalies, psychomotor delay, failure to thrive, and skin abnormalities	Gene panel for RASopathies
Constitutional mismatch repair deficiency syndrome	MLH1, MSH2, MSH6, PMS2, EPCAM (AR)	Adenomatous colonic polyps, multiple malignancies including colonic adenocarcinoma, glioblastoma, medulloblastoma, lymphoma, and a positive family history of Lynch syndrome-associated malignancies on both sides of the family	Gene panel for Lynch syndrome genes
Multiple café-au-lait spots	N/A (AD)	6 or more CALMs in multiple generations without NF1-associated features	No genetic testing available
Familial progressive hyper and hypopigmentation syndrome	KITLG (AR)	Progressive, diffuse, partly blotchy hyperpigmented lesions with scattered hypopigmented spots and lentigines	KITLG gene testing
Fanconi anemia	FANCA and other genes (AR)	Faint ill-defined CALMs "shadow spots," hypopigmented macules, skinfold frecklelike macules, progressive bone marrow failure, short stature, hypogonadism, thumb or other radial ray abnormalities, and skeletal malformations	DNA breakage studies Gene panel for bone marrow failure syndromes

(continued on next page)

Table 2
(continued)

Condition	Gene (Inheritance)	Associated Features[a]	Additional Testing to Consider
Legius syndrome	SPRED1 (AD)	6 or more CALMs, intertriginous freckling, lipomas, macrocephaly, and learning disabilities	SPRED1 gene testing
Noonan syndrome with lentigines	PTPN11 (AD)	Small brown lentigines, café noir spots, CALMs, dysmorphic facial features, obstructive cardiomyopathy, pulmonary stenosis, growth abnormalities, and sensorineural hearing loss	PTPN11 gene testing
McCune-Albright syndrome	GNAS (Sporadic)	Coast of Maine CALMs associated with the lines of Blaschko, fibrous dysplasia, and endocrinopathies	GNAS gene testing from affected tissue (not blood)
Neurofibromatosis type 1	NF1 (AD)	6 or more CALMs, skinfold freckling, neurofibromas, plexiform neurofibromas, Lisch nodules, optic gliomas, skeletal dysplasia, macrocephaly, nevus anemicus, and juvenile xanthogranuloma	NF1 gene testing (DNA) ± RNA sequencing
Neurofibromatosis type 2	NF2 (AD)	Schwannomas, cutaneous plaques with hypertrichosis, light irregularly bordered CALMs, subcutaneous nodular tumors, peripheral neuropathy, and ophthalmologic lesions	NF2 gene testing (DNA) ± RNA sequencing
Noonan syndrome	PTPN11, SOS2, and other genes (AD)	Skin hyperlaxity, easy bruising, keratosis pilaris, temporal alopecia, distinctive facial features, developmental delay, learning difficulties, short stature, congenital heart disease, renal anomalies, lymphatic malformations	Gene panel for RASopathies
Piebaldism	KIT (AD)	Hypopigmented patches of skin and hair, hyperpigmentation of skin, CALMs, and axillary/inguinal freckling	KIT gene testing
PTEN hamartoma tumor syndrome	PTEN (AD)	Hamartomas, trichilemmomas, papillomatous papule, acral and plantar keratoses, lipomas, autism spectrum disorder, and macrocephaly	PTEN gene testing

(continued on next page)

Table 2
(continued)

Condition	Gene (Inheritance)	Associated Features[a]	Additional Testing to Consider
Ring chromosome syndrome 7, 11, 12, 15, and 17	Sporadic	Depends on which chromosome but may include CALMs, nevus flammeus, dark pigmented nevi, patchy hypopigmented areas, microcephaly, mental delay, short stature, and skeletal abnormalities	Karyotype
RSS	11p15 locus Chromosome 7 (Sporadic) CDKN1C, IGF2, PLAGL2, HMGA2 (AD)	Growth restriction, relative macrocephaly, craniofacial abnormalities, mild cognitive impairment, and delay	Molecular and methylation testing of 11p15 and uniparental disomy 7 ± RSS gene panel testing
Tuberous sclerosis	TSC1, TSC2 (AD)	Facial angiofibromas, ash leaf macules, thumbprintlike macules, confettilike skin lesions, shagreen patch, Koenen tumors, hamartomas, multisystem lymphangioleiomyomatosis, epilepsy, cognitive deficits	TSC1 and TSC2 gene testing

Abbreviations: AD, autosomal dominant; AFP, Alpha fetoprotein; AR, autosomal recessive; *ATM*, ataxia telangiectasia mutated gene; *BRAF*, B-RAF proto-oncogene; *CDKN1C*, cyclin-dependent kinase inhibitor 1C; EPCAM, epithelial cell adhesion molecule; *FANCA*, FA complementation group A; *GNAS*, GNAS complex locus; *HMGA2*, high mobility group AT-hook 2; *IFG2*, insulinlike growth factor 2; *KIT*, KIT proto-oncogene receptor tyrosine kinase; *KITLG*, KIT ligand; serine/threonine kinase, *MAP2K1/2*; mitogen-activated protein kinase kinase 1, *MLH1*; MutL, *Escherichia coli* homolog of 1, *MSH2*; MutS, *E coli* homolog of 2, *MSH6*; *MutS, E coli* homolog of 6; NF1, neurofibromin 1; *NF2*, neurofibromin 2; *PLAGL2*, PLAG1 like zinc finger 2; *PTEN*, phosphate and tensin homolog; , *PMS2*, postmeiotic segregation increased *Saccharomyces cerevisiae* 2; *PTPN11*, protein tyrosine phosphatase nonreceptor type 11; RSS, Russel-Silver syndrome; *SPRED 1*, sprouty-related EVH1 domain-containing protein 1; *SOS2*, SOS RAS/RAC guanine nucleotide exchange factor 2; *TSC1*, TSC1 gene; *TSC2*, TSC2 gene.
[a] All disorders listed have had multiple CALMs associated with them.

methods develop. Furthermore, the VUS status can be reviewed every 2 years for reclassification.

Further genetic testing might be warranted for other genetic conditions like Noonan syndrome with lentigines or Constitutional mismatch repair deficiency (CMMRD) depending on the clinical picture and family history. Referral to Clinical Genetics can be considered if a rarer syndromic disorder associated with CALMs is suspected.

CAFÉ AU LAIT MACULES NOT MEETING THE NEUROFIBROMATOSIS TYPE 1 NATIONAL INSTITUTES OF HEALTH CRITERIA

For patients presenting with less than 6 CALMs or with CALMs smaller than 5 or 15 mm, in the prepubertal and postpubertal stages, respectively, the diagnosis of NF1 becomes less likely.

Furthermore, it is important to remember that 1 to 3 CALMs with no underlying association is common in the general population.[57] For very young patients with less than 6 CALMs that lack other clinical features or family history of NF1, clinical follow-up is recommended to monitor for the apparition of additional CALMs or others NF1 features.[2] In older children who are otherwise healthy and present with less than 6 CALMs, they do not warrant follow-up for the skin change alone. Individuals with 6 or more CALMs not meeting the size requirement of the NIH criteria can be monitored annually for NF1-related features until at least 6 years old.

As was highlighted, atypical CALMs are associated with NF1 if there are 6 or more, but the risk is lower than with typical CALMs.[2,3] Clinical follow-up is appropriate for patients with 6 or more

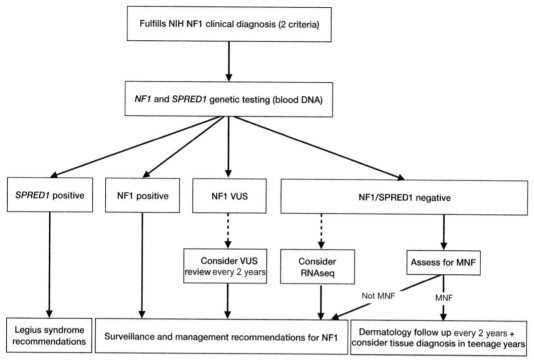

Fig. 6. Approach to the genetic diagnosis of NF1 if meeting more than 1 NF1 NIH criteria. RNAseq, RNA sequencing; SPRED1, sprouty-related EVH1 domain-containing 1; VUS, variant of unknown significance.

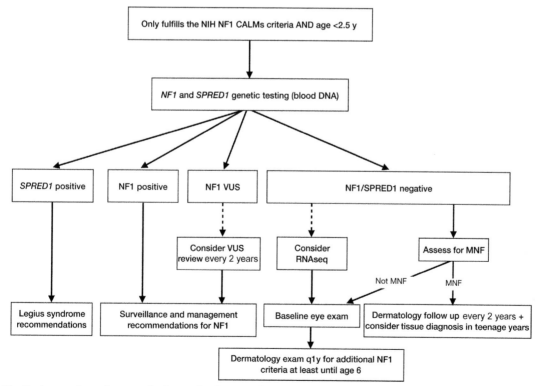

Fig. 7. Approach to the genetic diagnosis of young children who solely meet the CALMs' NIH criteria. RNAseq, RNA sequencing; SPRED1, sprouty-related EVH1 domain-containing 1; VUS, variant of unknown significance.

atypical CALMs, and NF1 or Legius syndrome should be considered. Other genetic diseases could be considered if there are less than 6 atypical CALMs. Genetic testing can be helpful in the diagnostic process if uncertainty is high.

OTHER CLUES FROM HISTORY AND PHYSICAL EXAMINATION

On history, it is important to enquire about a family history of genetic conditions and CALMs. A family history of childhood cancers, Lynch syndrome cancers, or consanguinity could suggest an underlying inherited genetic disorder. A personal or familial history of neurodevelopmental challenges can also raise the suspicion for NF1 because developmental delay, speech delays, attention-deficit/hyperactivity disorder (particularly inattention), and autism spectrum disorder have been reported in patients with NF1.[58–60] Headaches, seizures, constipation, and midgastric abdominal pain have also been reported to be more common in patients with NF1.[12]

On physical examination, full physical examination with particular attention to detailed dermatologic and skeletal assessment is required to look for NF1 features based on the NIH criteria such as neurofibromas and osseous lesions. Optic gliomas can be assessed initially by examining visual acuity and looking for precocious puberty. A slit lamp examination is required to assess for Lisch nodules or choroidal abnormalities. Although not diagnostic criteria, other clues include macrocephaly, scoliosis, and short stature for age.[61] Juvenile xanthogranuloma (JXG) and nevus anemicus have been reported in 10% and 51% of patients with NF1, respectively.[62,63] Some experts argued for the inclusion of JXG and nevus anemicus in the NIH diagnostic criteria.[64] Pediatric hypertension occurs in approximately 4.2% of the NF1 population.[11] This number is higher than in the general pediatric population and is often related to vascular lesions like renal artery stenosis, aortic stenosis, and coarctation.[65]

THE IMPORTANCE OF EARLY DIAGNOSIS

Early recognition and diagnosis of a neurocutaneous disease such as NF1 leads to improved outcomes and allows for monitoring and treatment of associated complications.[12,66] As well, new therapies are emerging for the treatment of optic gliomas, plexiform neurofibromas, and peripheral nerve sheath tumors.[67] The health surveillance and management recommendations of patients with NF1 have been detailed in the review by Miller and colleagues (2019).[12] In addition, making a diagnosis of NF1 is important for families because it provides closure, the opportunity for anticipatory guidance for the affected individuals, and also informs the risk of NF1 in other family members or future offspring. A molecular NF1 diagnosis is essential to enable the option of reproductive planning and management. Furthermore, children with NF1 might have trouble communicating some of the complications of NF1 like optic gliomas (poor visual acuity) because of their age and CALMs may be the only presenting sign.[68] Finally, although limited right now, genotype-phenotype correlations will likely expand opportunities for personalized management in the future with ongoing research and advancement in genetics and genomics.[69]

SUMMARY

Although CALMs are common in the general population and are themselves benign, they can be the first and often only sign of an underlying genetic disease, especially in young children. Using the number, size, shape, and distribution of CALMs can be a powerful clinical tool in identifying children at risk of developing NF1. Care should be taken because significant overlap exists between CALMs-linked genetic diseases and misdiagnosing other hyperpigmented lesions as CALMs is also common. Genetic testing can be especially helpful in diagnosing NF1 when the presentation is atypical or the child is very young, although it might not be needed in all patients. In the absence of an alternative explanation for multiple CALMs, patients suspected of NF1 should be followed for the apparition of additional NF1 features regardless of genetic testing availability or outcomes.

CLINICS CARE POINTS

- One to 3 CALMs is a common finding in the general population and does not require further testing in the absence of other signs of neurocutaneous disease.

- Although NF1 is an autosomal dominant condition, a family history of NF1 is often absent because 50% of patients with NF1 have a de novo causative variant.

- Given the possibility of a missed *NF1* variant, a negative NF1 genetic test does not rule out NF1 and patients fulfilling clinical NIH diagnostic criteria for NF1 should follow NF1 management recommendations.

- Children younger than 2.5 years old who present with 6 or more CALMs should be genetically tested for *NF1* and *SPRED1* because these children have a high pretest probability of testing positive and thus benefiting from anticipatory guidance.

DISCLOSURE

The authors have nothing to disclose.

REFERENCES

1. Shah KN. The diagnostic and clinical significance of café-au-lait macules. Pediatr Clin North Am 2010; 57(5):1131–53.
2. Nunley KS, Gao F, Albers AC, et al. Predictive value of café au lait macules at initial consultation in the diagnosis of neurofibromatosis type 1. Arch Dermatol 2009;145(8):883–7.
3. Ben-Shachar S, Dubov T, Toledano-Alhadef H, et al. Predicting neurofibromatosis type 1 risk among children with isolated café-au-lait macules. J Am Acad Dermatol 2017;76(6):1077–83.e3.
4. Ruggiero JL, Dodds M, Freese R, et al. Cutaneous findings in Fanconi Anemia. J Am Acad Dermatol 2020. https://doi.org/10.1016/j.jaad.2020.08.047.
5. Alper JC, Holmes LB. The incidence and significance of birthmarks in a cohort of 4,641 newborns. Pediatr Dermatol 1983;1(1):58–68.
6. Riccardi VM. Neurofibromatosis and Albright's syndrome. Dermatol Clin 1987;5(1):193–203.
7. Rivers JK, MacLennan R, Kelly JW, et al. The Eastern Australian childhood nevus study: prevalence of atypical nevi, congenital nevus-like nevi, and other pigmented lesions. J Am Acad Dermatol 1995;32(6):957–63.
8. Williams VC, Lucas J, Babcock MA, et al. Neurofibromatosis type 1 revisited. Pediatrics 2009; 123(1):124–33.
9. McLean DI, Gallagher RP. "Sunburn" freckles, café-au-lait macules, and other pigmented lesions of schoolchildren: The Vancouver Mole Study. J Am Acad Dermatol 1995;32(4):565–70.
10. Tekin M, Bodurtha JN, Riccardi VM. Café au lait spots: the pediatrician's perspective. Pediatr Rev 2001;22(3):82–90.
11. Friedman JM, Birch PH. Type 1 neurofibromatosis: a descriptive analysis of the disorder in 1,728 patients. Am J Med Genet 1997;70(2):138–43.
12. Miller DT, Freedenberg D, Schorry E, et al. Health supervision for children with neurofibromatosis type 1. Pediatrics 2019;143(5):e20190660.
13. Lammert M, Friedman JM, Kluwe L, et al. Prevalence of neurofibromatosis 1 in German children at elementary school enrollment. Arch Dermatol 2005; 141(1):71–4.
14. Littler M, Morton NE. Segregation analysis of peripheral neurofibromatosis (NF1). J Med Genet 1990; 27(5):307–10.
15. National Institutes of Health Consensus Development Conference Statement: neurofibromatosis. Bethesda, Md., USA, July 13-15, 1987. Neurofibromatosis 1988; 1(3):172-8.
16. Gutmann DH, Aylsworth A, Carey JC, et al. The diagnostic evaluation and multidisciplinary management of neurofibromatosis 1 and neurofibromatosis 2. J Am Med Assoc 1997. https://doi.org/10.1001/jama.278.1.51.
17. DeBella K, Szudek J, Friedman JM. Use of the National Institutes of Health criteria for diagnosis of neurofibromatosis 1 in children. Pediatrics 2000; 105(3):608–14.
18. Tonsgard JH. Clinical manifestations and management of neurofibromatosis type 1. Semin Pediatr Neurol 2006;13(1):2–7.
19. Ward BA, Gutmann DH. Neurofibromatosis 1: from lab bench to clinic. Pediatr Neurol 2005;32(4):221–8.
20. Korf BR. Diagnostic outcome in children with multiple cafe au lait spots. Pediatrics 1992;90(6):924–7.
21. Messiaen LM, Callens T, Mortier G, et al. Exhaustive mutation analysis of the NF1 gene allows identification of 95% of mutations and reveals a high frequency of unusual splicing defects. Hum Mutat 2000;15(6):541–55.
22. Upadhyaya M, Huson SM, Davies M, et al. An absence of cutaneous neurofibromas associated with a 3-bp inframe deletion in exon 17 of the NF1 gene (c.2970-2972 delAAT): evidence of a clinically significant NF1 genotype-phenotype correlation. Am J Hum Genet 2007;80(1):140–51.
23. Legius E, Messiaen L, Wolkenstein P, et al. Revised diagnostic criteria for neurofibromatosis type 1 and Legius syndrome: an international consensus recommendation. Genet Med 2021;19:1–8.
24. Wimmer K, Yao S, Claes K, et al. Spectrum of single- and multiexon NF1 copy number changes in a cohort of 1,100 unselected NF1 patients. Genes Chromosom Cancer 2006;45(3):265–76.
25. Ruggieri M, Huson SM. The clinical and diagnostic implications of mosaicism in the neurofibromatoses. Neurology 2001;56(11):1433–43.
26. Maertens O, De Schepper S, Vandesompele J, et al. Molecular dissection of isolated disease features in mosaic neurofibromatosis type 1. Am J Hum Genet 2007;81(2):243–51.
27. Wolkenstein P, Mahmoudi A, Zeller J, et al. More on the frequency of segmental neurofibromatosis. Arch Dermatol 1995;131(12):1465.
28. García-Romero MT, Parkin P, Lara-Corrales I. Mosaic neurofibromatosis Type 1: a systematic review. Pediatr Dermatol 2016;33:9–17.

29. Tanito K, Ota A, Kamide R, et al. Clinical features of 58 Japanese patients with mosaic neurofibromatosis 1. J Dermatol 2014;41(8):724–8.

30. Ejerskov C, Farholt S, Skovby F, et al. Clinical presentations of 23 half-siblings from a mosaic neurofibromatosis type 1 sperm donor. Clin Genet 2016; 89(3):346–50.

31. Messiaen L, Yao S, Brems H, et al. Clinical and mutational spectrum of neurofibromatosis type 1-like syndrome. JAMA 2009;302(19):2111–8.

32. Brems H, Chmara M, Sahbatou M, et al. Germline loss-of-function mutations in SPRED1 cause a neurofibromatosis 1-like phenotype. Nat Genet 2007;39(9):1120–6.

33. Pasmant E, Gilbert-Dussardier B, Petit A, et al. SPRED1, a RAS MAPK pathway inhibitor that causes Legius syndrome, is a tumour suppressor downregulated in paediatric acute myeloblastic leukaemia. Oncogene 2015;34(5):631–8.

34. Allanson JE. Noonan syndrome. J Med Genet 1987; 24(1):9–13.

35. Sarkozy A, Conti E, Digilio MC, et al. Clinical and molecular analysis of 30 patients with multiple lentigines LEOPARD syndrome. J Med Genet 2004; 41(5):e68.

36. Tidyman WE, Rauen KA. Noonan, Costello and cardio-facio-cutaneous syndromes: dysregulation of the Ras-MAPK pathway. Expert Rev Mol Med 2008;10:e37.

37. Siegel DH, McKenzie J, Frieden IJ, et al. Dermatological findings in 61 mutation-positive individuals with cardiofaciocutaneous syndrome. Br J Dermatol 2011;164(3):521–9.

38. Zhang J, Li M, Yao Z. Molecular screening strategies for NF1-like syndromes with café-au-lait macules (Review). Mol Med Rep 2016;14(5):4023–9.

39. Chiu YE, Dugan S, Basel D, et al. Association of piebaldism, multiple café-au-lait macules, and intertriginous freckling: clinical evidence of a common pathway between KIT and sprouty-related, Ena/vasodilator-stimulated phosphoprotein homology-1 domain containing protein 1 (SPRED1). Pediatr Dermatol 2013;30(3):379–82.

40. Zhang J, Cheng R, Liang J, et al. Report of a child with sporadic familial progressive hyper- and hypopigmentation caused by a novel KITLG mutation. Br J Dermatol 2016;175(6):1369–71.

41. Lalor L, Davies OMT, Basel D, et al. Café au lait spots: when and how to pursue their genetic origins. Clin Dermatol 2020. https://doi.org/10.1016/j.clindermatol.2020.03.005.

42. Rotern V, Masouyé I, Delozier-Blanchet CD, et al. Cutaneous findings in ring chromosome 7 syndrome. Dermatology 1993;186(2):84–7.

43. Etzler J, Peyrl A, Zatkova A, et al. RNA-based mutation analysis identifies an unusual MSH6 splicing defect and circumvents PMS2 pseudogene interference. Hum Mutat 2008;29(2):299–305.

44. Greenberger S, Berkun Y, Ben-Zeev B, et al. Dermatologic manifestations of ataxia-telangiectasia syndrome. J Am Acad Dermatol 2013;68(6):932–6.

45. Mautner VF, Lindenau M, Baser ME, et al. Skin abnormalities in neurofibromatosis 2. Arch Dermatol 1997;133(12):1539–43.

46. Evans DGR, Huson SM, Donnai D, et al. A clinical study of Type 2 neurofibromatosis. Q J Med 1992; 84(1):603–18.

47. Ruggieri M, Iannetti P, Polizzi A, et al. Earliest clinical manifestations and natural history of neurofibromatosis type 2 (NF2) in childhood: a study of 24 patients. Neuropediatrics 2005;36(1):21–34.

48. Mccune DJ. Osteitis fibrosa cystica : the case of a nine year old girl who also exhibits precocious puberty, multiple pigmentation of the skin and hyperthyroidism. Am J Dis Child 1936;52:743–4.

49. Rieger E, Kofler R, Borkenstein M, et al. Melanotic macules following Blaschko's lines in McCune-Albright syndrome. Br J Dermatol 1994;130(2):215–20.

50. Benedict PH, Szabó G, Fitzpatrick TB, et al. Melanotic Macules in Albright's syndrome and in neurofibromatosis. JAMA 1968;205(9):618–26.

51. Cardis MA, Deklotz CMC. Cutaneous manifestations of tuberous sclerosis complex and the paediatrician's role. Arch Dis Child 2017;102(9):858–63.

52. Jóźwiak S, Schwartz RA, Janniger CK, et al. Skin lesions in children with tuberous sclerosis complex: Their prevalence, natural course, and diagnostic significance. Int J Dermatol 1998;37(12):911–7.

53. Charrow J, Listernick R, Ward K. Autosomal dominant multiple cafe-au-lait spots and neurofibromatosis-1: evidence of non-linkage. Am J Med Genet 1993;45(5):606–8.

54. Abeliovich D, Gelman-Kohan Z, Silverstein S, et al. Familial café au lait spots: a variant of neurofibromatosis type 1. J Med Genet 1995;32(12):985–6.

55. OMIM Entry - 114030 - Cafe-au-lait spots, multiple. Available at: https://omim.org/entry/114030. Accessed July 24, 2021.

56. Yao R, Wang L, Yu Y, et al. Diagnostic value of multiple café-au-lait macules for neurofibromatosis 1 in Chinese children. J Dermatol 2016. https://doi.org/10.1111/1346-8138.13169.

57. Landau M, Krafchik BR. The diagnostic value of cafe-au-lait macules. J Am Acad Dermatol 1999; 40(6 I):877–90.

58. Thompson HL, Viskochil DH, Stevenson DA, et al. Speech-language characteristics of children with neurofibromatosis type 1. Am J Med Genet A 2010;152(2):284–90.

59. Garg S, Green J, Leadbitter K, et al. Neurofibromatosis type 1 and autism spectrum disorder. Pediatrics 2013;132(6):e1642.

60. Coud FX, Mignot C, Lyonnet S, et al. Early grade repetition and inattention associated with neurofibromatosis type 1. J Atten Disord 2007;11(2):101–5.

61. Clementi M, Milani S, Mammi I, et al. Neurofibromatosis type I growth charts. Am J Med Genet 1999; 87(4):317–23.

62. Ferrari F, Masurel A, Olivier-Faivre L, et al. Juvenile xanthogranuloma and nevus anemicus in the diagnosis of neurofibromatosis type 1. JAMA Dermatol 2014;150(1):42–6.

63. Marque M, Roubertie A, Jaussent A, et al. Nevus anemicus in neurofibromatosis type 1: a potential new diagnostic criterion. J Am Acad Dermatol 2013;69(5):768–75.

64. Tadini G, Milani D, Menni F, et al. Is it time to change the neurofibromatosis 1 diagnostic criteria? Eur J Intern Med 2014;25(6):506–10.

65. Friedman JM, Arbiter J, Epstein JA, et al. Cardiovascular disease in neurofibromatosis 1: Report of the NF1 Cardiovascular Task Force. Genet Med 2002; 4(3):105–11.

66. Bergqvist C, Servy A, Valeyrie-Allanore L, et al. Neurofibromatosis 1 French national guidelines based on an extensive literature review since 1966. Orphanet J Rare Dis 2020;15(1):1–23.

67. Gross AM, Dombi E, Widemann BC. Current status of MEK inhibitors in the treatment of plexiform neurofibromas. Child's Nerv Syst 2020;36(10):2443–52.

68. Blazo MA, Lewis RA, Chintagumpala MM, et al. Outcomes of systematic screening for optic pathway tumors in children with Neurofibromatosis Type 1. Am J Med Genet 2004;127A(3):224–9.

69. Kehrer-Sawatzki H, Mautner VF, Cooper DN. Emerging genotype–phenotype relationships in patients with large NF1 deletions. Hum Genet 2017; 136(4):349–76.

Pigmented Lesions in Children
Update on Clinical, Histopathologic and Ancillary Testing

Diana Bartenstein Reusch, MD[a], Elena B. Hawryluk, MD, PhD[b,c],*

KEYWORDS

- Congenital melanocytic nevus • Atypical spitz tumor • Pediatric melanoma

KEY POINTS

- Congenital melanocytic nevi confer a risk of melanoma that is influenced by size and the number of nevi.
- Early screening of appropriate patients can provide insight regarding melanoma risk.
- Spitzoid proliferations in the pediatric population generally follow a banal clinical course; molecular studies have not yet been validated in this age group.
- Melanoma can present diversely in the pediatric population compared with adults.

INTRODUCTION

Patients are commonly referred to pediatric dermatology for evaluation of pigmented lesions. For families, pediatricians, and dermatologists alike, malignancy is the main fear. An evolving body of literature is available to inform diagnosis and management. In this article, we provide an update on the clinical, histopathologic, and ancillary testing for 3 categories of particularly challenging pigmented lesions: congenital melanocytic nevi (CMN), spitzoid neoplasms, and pediatric melanoma.

CONGENITAL MELANOCYTIC NEVI

CMN are pigmented proliferations that may be observed either at birth or within the first few weeks of life. The estimated incidence varies, but is generally reported at less than 6%.[1] Among all CMN, smaller birthmarks are much more common than larger lesions (**Fig. 1**). The overall incidence increases when tardive CMN are also accounted for. Tardive CMN, which are sometimes referred to as congenital nevus-like nevi, present within the first few years of life and may be clinically, dermoscopically, and histologically indistinguishable from earlier onset CMN.[2,3] Research is underway to elucidate the origin of CMN cells, because many hypotheses for development exist[4,5]

A careful clinical inspection of CMN can inform expectations regarding a child's risk of developing malignant melanoma and central nervous system involvement, which includes neurocutaneous melanosis or neurocutaneous melanocytosis, as well as other pathologies. The term "congenital melanocytic nevus syndrome" has been proposed for children with CMN in addition to extracutaneous features. Mosaic postzygotic mutation of *NRAS* underlies many CMN and associated central nervous system changes.[6] It has been noted that some children with larger and multiple CMN possess certain facial characteristics, such as a prominent forehead and long philtrum, and it has been proposed that these features also be considered syndromic.[7]

[a] Harvard Combined Dermatology Residency Training Program, 50 Staniford Street, Suite 200, Boston, MA 02114, USA; [b] Department of Dermatology, Massachusetts General Hospital, 50 Staniford Street, Suite 200, Boston, MA 02114, USA; [c] Dermatology Section, Boston Children's Hospital, Harvard Medical School, Boston, MA 02115, USA
* Corresponding author.
E-mail address: ehawryluk@mgh.harvard.edu

Dermatol Clin 40 (2022) 25–36
https://doi.org/10.1016/j.det.2021.09.003

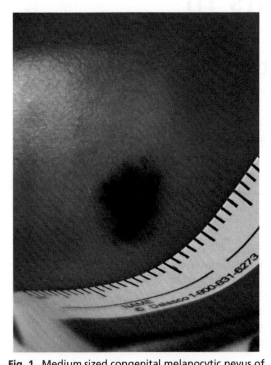

Fig. 1. Medium sized congenital melanocytic nevus of the chin on a child.

When evaluating a patient with CMN, it is important to assess for size, satellite or multiple nevi, and evolution. Imaging, histopathology, and genetic testing can also be helpful in selected circumstances, as detailed elsewhere in this article.

Clinical Assessment

Size
The classification of CMN is based on measurement by projected adult size,[8] with groupings as follows:

- Small CMN: less than 1.5 cm
- Medium CMN: 1.5–20.0 cm
- Large CMN: greater than 20–40 cm
- Giant CMN: greater than 40 cm

Measuring the CMN size is important for risk stratification. As CMN size increases, so too does melanoma risk. In a comprehensive review of the literature from 1966 to 2011, it was found that the incidence of melanoma in patients with a CMN greater than 20 cm (large and giant CMNs) was approximately 2%.[9] In a recent prospective cohort, 8% of patients with a CMN greater than 60 cm developed melanoma, whereas melanoma incidence remained at 1% for all other patients.[10] Notably, there is variability between reported results, and patients with giant CMN and many satellites remain at greatest risk with upwards of 10%

to 15% risk of melanoma.[11,12] Patients with small and medium sized CMN may have a mildly increased risk of developing melanoma, but previous calculations have likely been skewed by the largest of lesions in heterogenous cohorts.

For benign appearing, clinically stable CMN of all sizes, we recommend conservative monitoring. All patients should be taught to inspect and palpate their birthmarks routinely. For patients with a CMN greater than 20 cm (**Fig. 2**), dermatologists can additionally monitor patients using photographs and dermoscopy.

A biopsy for histopathologic analysis may be considered if evolution concerning for melanoma occurs. Warning signs include ulceration, pain, rapid growth, and other unexpected evolution.[13] However, whereas it was historically recommended to excise each and every CMN, this practice is no longer the standard of care.[14] Malignant degeneration is quite uncommon in small and medium CMN and excision does not seem to decrease the risk of melanoma for patients with large or giant CMNs. Excision, which may cause substantial morbidity and suboptimal cosmetic results, does not prevent melanoma from occurring in other cutaneous sites, underneath skin grafts, or internally.[11] It remains to be determined whether providers have an easier time detecting melanoma that develops in preintervention versus postintervention skin, but anecdotally, it can be challenging to evaluate for malignant transformation in patients who have undergone serial excisions, dermabrasion, and skin grafts. Families should be counseled extensively about the risks and benefits of any invasive intervention before pursuing treatment.

Satellite and multiple nevi
Many patients with large and giant CMN have small CMN surrounding their largest lesion. Customary terminology designates these smaller CMN as "satellite nevi," and the presence or absence of satellite nevi has been evaluated as a prognostic factor for the development of CMN complications. However, it has alternatively been proposed that classification of CMN as single versus multiple (>1 CMN regardless of size and configuration) may be more appropriate.[15] The presence of multiple CMNs is a risk factor for the development of melanoma, central nervous system involvement, and adverse outcomes, regardless of configuration.[9]

Location
Historically, CMN in a posterior axial distribution were thought to be associated with neurocutaneous melanosis and adverse outcomes.[16] It is now

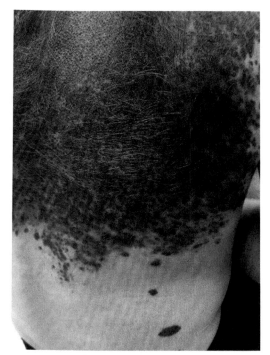

Fig. 2. Large congenital melanocytic nevus of the torso on a child.

questioned, however, whether an axial location for large and giant CMN simply represents the most common site of involvement without independently portending a poor prognosis.[12]

Evolution

During early infancy, a CMN may grow rapidly.[17] In childhood, it is expected that a CMN will grow proportionally as a child grows. It is also common for CMN to develop changes in thickness, texture, hair growth, and color over time. Although some CMN darken, others substantially lighten without treatment.

Benign proliferative nodules and neuroid overgrowth may be present at birth in large and giant CMN, or develop later in childhood. There are variable clinical presentations for these nonmalignant growths and reassuring features include a soft or slightly firm texture, multiple nodules, a lack of ulceration, and stability after an initial period of growth.[10,18]

Of course, any change in a CMN must be scrutinized so as to not miss malignant degeneration. If there are no red flag signs warranting excision at the initial evaluation (eg, rock hard texture, ulceration, or associated lymphadenopathy), providers may follow Kinsler and colleagues'[10] algorithm for the management of new bumps noticed within a patient's CMN:

1. Complete a thorough clinical examination that is documented with high-quality photography.
2. Reassess the patient in 4 weeks.
   a. If the CMN is unchanged, continue regular monitoring until the provider is assured of lesional stability.
   b. If the lesion has changed or if any red flag signs develop, perform an excisional biopsy for further characterization.

Ancillary Testing

MRI

MRI is the preferred modality to screen for central nervous system involvement in patients with CMN. MRI screening of the central nervous system (brain and spine) should be considered for the following patient groups:

1. Infants with 2 or more CMN (of any size)[19]
2. Infants with large or giant CMN (>20 cm)
3. Any patient who demonstrates neurologic change (in the context of any sized CMN)

Patients with multiple as well as large or giant CMN are at an increased risk of central nervous system abnormality, whether owing to melanocytic proliferation or other process; risk increases as size and number increases.[19] Alternative guidelines proposed by Krengel and Marghoob recommend central nervous system imaging for the following patient groups only[20]:

1. Patients with giant CMN greater than 40 cm
2. Patients with multiple medium CMN
3. Patients with multiple satellite nevi
4. Any patient with a concerning neurologic change

An MRI of the full central nervous system is ideally performed for high-risk patients within the first 6 months of life, before myelination occurs, and an when MRI can be performed without general anesthesia using the "swaddle and bottle" approach, to serve as a baseline. After initial imaging, or if imaging is not pursued, routine clinical monitoring for neurologic changes should be performed by the patient's pediatrician and dermatologist. Abnormal neurologic signs or symptoms should prompt repeat MRI and referral to neurology.

In 1 prospective study, on baseline imaging, high-risk patients with CMN were found to have intraparenchymal melanosis as well as other central nervous system pathology, including but not limited to cysts, tumors, and white matter changes.[19] Whereas the MRI finding of intraparenchymal melanosis was associated with seizures and neurodevelopmental abnormalities, it seemed to carry a low risk of central nervous system melanoma; this finding is in contrast with the increased risk of melanoma observed in association with other central nervous system abnormalities identified on baseline imaging.[19] As data emerge, our understanding of neurocutaneous melanosis continues to evolve. Parents must be counseled that individual management and outcomes are unique for each patient. Central nervous system findings on a baseline scan are neither fully predictive nor prognostic; rather, they provide clinicians with additional information that will inform overall surveillance and management.

Histopathology

CMN are diagnosed clinically and sampling for histopathology is typically reserved for evaluation of lumps and bumps that grow within a CMN, for example, to distinguish benign proliferative nodule from melanoma. Differentiating these diagnoses can be challenging for dermatopathologists because it is not uncommon to see mitoses, atypia, and other traditionally concerning features in benign CMN growths.[18] Further research is underway, but it has been proposed that ulceration, high-grade nuclear atypia, and high mitotic counts may be particularly concerning for melanoma when arising in an expansile nodule of epithelioid cells, as opposed to a small round blue cell or complex pattern.[18] For these challenging lesions, it is important to have an experienced dermatopathologist reviewing the patient's slides. Genetic testing can also provide key information.

Genetic testing

Most CMN result from postzygotic NRAS and BRAF gene mutations,[21] and mosaic NRAS expression is responsible for the majority of patients with multiple CMN, large CMN, and/or neurocutaneous melanosis.[6,21] Our current understanding is that additional mutations are required for malignant transformation. Therefore, for patients with CMN, molecular diagnostics can help to inform evaluation of benign proliferative nodule versus malignant melanoma. Fluorescence in situ hybridization (FISH) and comparative genomic hybridization can demonstrate copy number gains and losses, which may occur in both benign and malignant lesions, but are typically thought to be more concerning if partial as opposed to full chromosomes are affected.[18] Hotspot genotyping is another adjunctive tool that may be used to evaluate for melanoma, because multiple foci of melanoma within a patient with CMN patient may demonstrate the same mutation and provide distinction from proliferative nodules. NRAS hotspot mutations have been identified in

patients with CMN who suffered from fatal melanoma, and BRAF hotspot genotyping can also be used.[22]

CLINICS CARE POINTS

- Evaluating patients with CMN by the size and number of CMN is important for risk stratification. CMN greater than 60 cm and multiple CMN confer an unambiguously increased risk for melanoma and central nervous system disease.
- For CMN of all sizes, clinical examination remains the gold standard for melanoma surveillance. Surgical excision is not recommended for primary malignancy prevention.
- Baseline imaging of the central nervous system should be obtained for high-risk patients.

SPITZ NEVI AND SPITZOID NEOPLASMS

Spitz nevi are epithelioid and spindled cell proliferations that were first identified and named ("benign juvenile melanoma") by Dr Sophie Spitz in 1948.[23] Since then, a spectrum from benign to malignant has been recognized and lesions are now classified on the spitzoid neoplasm spectrum as benign Spitz nevi, atypical Spitz tumors, or spitzoid melanomas (Fig. 3). Spitz melanoma is a subtype of spitzoid melanoma that is distinguished by the presence of typical kinase fusions or HRAS mutations, despite overlapping histopathologic features.[24]

Recommendations for the evaluation and management of adults with spitzoid tumors vary greatly from those for pediatric patients. Clinically banal appearing spitzoid lesions in adults carry significant risk, in contrast with pediatric lesions.[25] This article focuses on the care of children and adolescents only.

Identification

Benign, nonpigmented Spitz nevi present as pink to red papules that are symmetric, may be dome shaped, and are asymptomatic. They are typically less than 6 mm in size. At initial onset, they may undergo a period of rapid growth, but then achieve stability. Many lesions ultimately undergo involution.[26] Differential diagnosis includes vascular lesion, xanthogranuloma, and molluscum, although close clinical inspection can usually distinguish these entities.

Spitz nevi can also be pigmented. These lesions are brown to black and can be quite striking in fair-skinned patients. However, dermoscopic examination will reveal the classic starburst pattern,

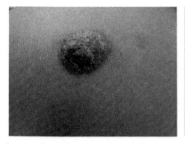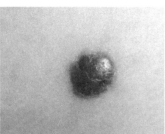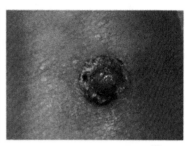

Fig. 3. Clinical appearance of pediatric typical Spitz nevus, atypical Spitz tumor, and spitzoid melanoma.[27] (*From* Bartenstein, D., Fisher, J., Stamoulis, C., Weldon, C., Huang, J., Gellis, S., Liang, M., Schmidt, B. and Hawryluk, E. (2019), Clinical features and outcomes of spitzoid proliferations in children and adolescents. Br J Dermatol, 181: 366–372.)

which is pathognomonic. Features suggestive of atypia or melanoma include persistent evolution, ulceration, bleeding, pain, and irritation of the surrounding skin.

Natural History and Clinical Outcomes

Traditionally, it has been thought that Spitz nevi do not carry malignant potential, atypical spitzoid tumors have uncertain risk, and malignant spitzoid melanoma can lead to a fatal outcome.[27] However, spitzoid tumors of all subtypes have yielded excellent outcomes in children and adolescents specifically. This factor is a key difference from the adult population.

In a survey study of pediatric dermatologists who had evaluated approximately 10,000 Spitz nevi and atypical Spitz tumors in their practices, no deaths were observed.[28] To date, the 2 largest retrospective cohorts for pediatric spitzoid neoplasms come from Boston Children's Hospital and Children's Hospital of Wisconsin.[29,30] Cumulatively, these cohorts capture 888 spitzoid lesions, without any known deaths occurring. There were 3 patients diagnosed with spitzoid melanomas at Boston Children's Hospital, the youngest of whom was 14.7 years. At Children's Hospital of Wisconsin, 1 spitzoid melanoma was diagnosed in a 10-year-old.

Although fatal outcome from a spitzoid tumor is exceedingly uncommon in pediatric patients, it has been reported,[31,32] and there is not sufficient evidence at present to forego standard melanoma treatment in those diagnosed with spitzoid melanoma. It is impossible to say whether favorable outcomes observed have been confounded by treatments received or publication bias.

Clinical Approach and Workup

For healthy patients who present with banal, typical appearing Spitz nevi, it is reasonable to clinically monitor the lesion with repeat evaluation at 1- to 3-month intervals. If the lesion achieves stability, monitoring can be spaced to a less frequent interval such as every 6 to 12 months.[33] If the lesion develops any concerning features such as ulceration, bleeding, asymmetric growth, pain, crust or persistent growth/change, a biopsy should be pursued. Asymmetric or unexpected growth in a 1- to 3-month interval, or growth out of proportion with the patient's growth, should prompt a biopsy for histopathologic confirmation.

Histopathology

Histopathology remains the gold standard for differentiating spitzoid tumor subtypes, although their evaluation can be exceedingly challenging. Spitzoid proliferations that are biopsied should undergo evaluation by a dermatopathologist who is an expert in pediatric pigmented lesions before any treatment decisions are made to avoid overdiagnosis and undue treatment morbidity.

Molecular testing

Molecular testing has gained traction for diagnosis of adult melanomas. Exciting research is underway to determine the best use of molecular tools to characterize Spitz spectrum tumors and in some cases, attempt to differentiate benign from malignant. For several approaches described elsewhere in this article, testing is reported in adult or mixed cohorts and has not been validated in children[34–36]; therefore, any results obtained must be interpreted with caution.

The demonstration of kinase fusion is useful to distinguish a Spitz spectrum tumor from non-Spitz pigmented lesion.

- Kinase fusions
  - The characterizing molecular feature of a Spitz tumor is kinase fusion, such as *ROS1*, *NTRK1*, *ALK*, *BRAF*, and *RET*.[37]
  - Although these genomic changes can help to distinguish Spitz tumors from mimickers, kinase fusions do not differentiate benign

from malignant spitzoid tumors owing to substantial overlap. In 1 study, kinase fusions were found in 55% of Spitz nevi, 56% of atypical Spitz tumors, and 39% of spitzoid melanomas.[37]

For patients with atypical Spitz tumors or spitzoid melanomas, molecular testing may provide investigational and supportive information to help guide management decisions; existing data are summarized here:

- Telomerase reverse transcriptase (*TERT*) promoter *(Tert-p)* mutations
  - Promoter mutations in the *TERT* gene are common in conventional adult melanomas.
  - In 1 study of atypical Spitz tumors (n = 23) and spitzoid melanomas (n = 33), which included children and adults, all 4 patients with identified *TERT-p* mutations died from metastatic disease.[38] Two were adults and 2 were adolescents, ages 11 and 14.[39] No patients in this cohort without the *TERT-p* mutation experienced death.
  - Although *TERT-p* mutations represent a promising area of future study, there is not yet sufficient data to rely on this marker as a reliable predictor of malignancy or outcome in pediatric patients with spitzoid neoplasms.
- FISH
  - FISH uses specialized probes to detect chromosomal aberrations.
  - In 2009, the original 4-probe FISH assay including *RREB1, MYB,* centromere 6, and *CCND1* was reported to have 86.7% sensitivity and 95.4% specificity in distinguishing benign nevi from melanoma.[40] However, this cohort was not pediatric specific.
  - In 2012, an enhanced FISH assay with higher sensitivity and specificity as well as better targeting of spitzoid melanoma was proposed. This assay included *RREB1, CCND1, C-MYC,* and *CDKN2A* and reported that homozygous 9p21 (*CKDN2A*) deletions were significantly associated with aggressive behavior in spitzoid tumors.[41,42] This cohort was not pediatric specific.
  - The first pediatric-specific Spitz cohort analyzed with FISH emerged from Italy in 2014. This retrospective study included 20 Spitz nevi and 50 atypical Spitz tumors in patients aged 18 years and younger.[35] Researchers found that the traditional 4-probe FISH was positive in 20% of Spitz nevi and 30% of atypical Spitz tumors, indicating

that this ancillary test was not capable of distinguishing spitzoid subtypes. A 9p21 FISH was performed on 37 atypical Spitz tumor cases, demonstrating homozygous deletion in 2 cases and heterozygous deletion in 3 cases. The only fatal case in this cohort occurred in a patient with an atypical Spitz tumor who had heterozygous 9p21 loss, indicating that homozygous 9p21 deletion was neither fully sensitive nor specific to predict spitzoid behavior in this pediatric cohort.

  - A larger, prospective pediatric study of spitzoid proliferations was published in 2017 that did find a significant association between homozygous 9p21 deletion and disease recurrence, though the signal was less strong than in adult patients.[34] Among 85 patients with follow-up data, 9 had homozygous 9p21 deletions including 2 patients with disease recurrence and/or distant metastasis.[34] Although this study suggests that homozygous 9p21 deletions may provide complementary information for management decisions, the sample size remains too low for widespread extrapolation and standard use in pediatric patient care.
- PReferentially expressed Antigen in MElanoma (PRAME)
  - PRAME can be detected by performing immunohistochemical analysis on formalin-fixed and paraffin-embedded tissue blocks. It is a noninvasive adjunct that has been developed to distinguish benign melanocytic lesions from malignant melanoma.[43] In a recent analysis of 35 spitzoid proliferations, PRAME performed poorly.[36] PRAME was expressed in 1 of 20 Spitz nevi, 1 of 13 atypical Spitz tumors, and 1 of 2 spitzoid melanomas, suggesting this tool is not helpful in the evaluation of spitzoid lesions.

Sentinel lymph node biopsy

Sentinel lymph node biopsy (SLNB) should be pursued only for patients diagnosed with spitzoid melanoma as a top-line diagnosis. However, given the excellent outcomes observed for preadolescent patients diagnosed with Spitz melanoma (even in the presence of positive sentinel nodes), individual clinicians and families must carefully weigh the risks and benefits of SLNB in this patient population. The implications of a positive test include consideration of completion lymph node dissection versus imaging of the lymph node basin and consideration of adjuvant medical treatment. If completion lymph node dissection is pursued, the patient undergoes a major surgery the with risk of permanent complications, such as lymphedema. Adjuvant medical therapy might include chemotherapy agents with substantial morbidity.

Historically, SLNB was additionally recommended for patients with atypical Spitz tumors, and positive SLNB outcome resulted in upgrading of lesional classification to that of Spitz melanoma. However, research has failed to demonstrate a prognostic or therapeutic benefit from this practice.[44,45] In a large cohort of children and adults, survival was 99% for patients with SLNB positive atypical Spitz tumors.[45] Histopathology remains sufficient for tumor classification.

Re-excision

It is not necessary to re-excise a biopsy-proven benign Spitz nevus given the excellent clinical outcomes, but shared-decision making should be used with a patient's family. Incompletely excised Spitz nevi can recur with atypia[29] and re-excision with the goal of complete removal may be pursued to avoid future diagnostic confusion. Whether a Spitz nevus is documented as fully or incompletely excised on initial biopsy, recurrent nevus phenomenon should be discussed with families given that margin evaluation is imperfect in standard histopathologic evaluation.

It is important to re-excise atypical Spitz tumors to fully evaluate lesional histopathology and to avoid potential future confusion and overtreatment of a recurrent lesion.

Patients with Spitz melanoma should undergo re-excision with standard melanoma margins and additional management as dictated by tumor features.

CLINICS CARE POINTS

- Conservative monitoring may be pursued for pediatric patients presenting with banal appearing Spitz nevi.
- If a biopsy is pursued, complete sampling is ideal and the specimen should be reviewed by a dermatopathologist experienced in pediatric pigmented lesions.
- Ancillary testing has not been validated for pediatric Spitz tumors. Although it may provide additional information in challenging cases, it should be interpreted with caution and in the context of all available data.
- Re-excision may be pursued for benign Spitz nevi on an individual basis. It is recommended for atypical Spitz tumors and spitzoid melanomas.

PEDIATRIC MELANOMA
Epidemiology

Melanoma is an exceedingly rare diagnosis in the pediatric population. It is estimated to occur in less than 6 per 1 million children and adolescents.[46] Its incidence increases with age and therefore for young children, the risk is even lower. Data from the Surveillance, Epidemiology and End Results database suggests that between 2000 and 2010, less than 1 per 1 million children under the age of 4 years was affected.[46] The incidence was highest for patients 15 to 19 years old, at more than 17 per million, although this rate seems to be decreasing with time, perhaps owing to an increased awareness about the importance of photoprotection.[46]

Risk factors for pediatric melanoma include excessive sun and indoor tanning exposure, genetic susceptibility, immunosuppression, prior cancer, and the presence of giant and/or multiple CMN.

Outcomes

Fortunately, fatal melanoma is quite uncommon. A multicenter, retrospective study characterized pediatric patients who experienced fatal outcomes from their melanoma.[47] Queries at 16 academic institutions between the years of 1994 and 2017 identified 38 fatal cases. Twenty-four percent were diagnosed before the age of 11 and 76% were diagnosed between the ages of 11 and 20. The average survival time after diagnosis was 35.0 ± 29.7 months. Among the 16 cases with reported subtypes, nodular was the most common (50%), followed by superficial spreading (31%), and spitzoid (19%). All 3 patients who died from their Spitz melanomas were diagnosed postpubertally (ages 13, 15, and 19 years).

Many melanoma studies have replicated the finding that a favorable outcome is inversely correlated with age.[29,47,48] It remains to be determined whether a distinct pathophysiology underlies adult and pediatric melanomas, and perhaps even between childhood and adolescent melanomas, and whether other factors are at play.

Identification

Pediatric patients tend to be diagnosed with thicker melanomas than adult patients[48] and delays in identification may be contributory. Pediatric melanoma often presents differently than adult melanoma. The conventional ABCDs (Asymmetry, Border irregularity, Color variegation, Diameter >6 mm) apply more frequently to lesions in postpubertal patients, whereas these detection criteria will miss a substantial subset of melanoma in prepubertal patients. For example, amelanotic lesions are common in young children, and may be mistaken for a benign lesion such as a wart or molluscum.[49,50]

Visual inspection

Pediatric-specific ABCD criteria, intended to be used in concert with standard melanoma detection strategies, have been proposed as follows[51]:

- A: amelanosis
- B: bleeding, bumps
- C: uniform color
- D: variable diameter, de novo development

A high index of suspicion is required to identify pediatric melanoma. At the end of the day, evolution is likely the most sensitive predictor (**Fig. 4**). If a parent presents to clinic with high anxiety and concern about a child's lesion that clinically seems to be benign, close monitoring is a reasonable approach. For lesions with questionable characteristics, after performing a close visual inspection, dermoscopic examination, measurement, and photography, the patient should be brought back to clinic within 1 to 3 months, depending on the clinician's level of concern. Whereas benign lesions demonstrate no change or subtle, symmetric growth, malignant lesions will display prominent changes that might include asymmetric advancement of a border edge, ulceration, or focal color change. With this approach, clinicians can be confident in their clinical assessment, parents are reassured, and children are saved from unnecessary biopsies.

Dermoscopy

Dermoscopy is a noninvasive tool that can aid in the diagnosis of atypical appearing melanocytic proliferations. The following dermoscopic findings should raise concern for the diagnosis of pediatric melanoma[52]:

- Irregular globules
- Atypical network
- Blue white veil
- Atypical vessels
- Negative network

Additionally, the dermoscopic findings of atypical vessels and shiny white structures in amelanotic lesions may be red flags for spitzoid melanoma (**Fig. 5**).[52] For pigmented Spitz nevi, the classic starburst pattern is benign (**Fig. 6**), but other findings may indicate malignancy including black, blue-gray, and dark brown colors, a well as peripheral streaks and dark blotches.[52]

Melanoma Subtypes

Pediatric melanoma subtypes differ in their demographics, characteristics, risk factors and clinical course. A brief review is included, with asterisks representing the most common subtypes.

- *Conventional melanoma
  - Older teenagers are most likely to develop the same types of melanomas that develop in adults, including melanoma in situ, superficial spreading, and nodular subtypes. These melanomas often display single nucleotide variations consistent with UV damage, *BRAF* V600 activating mutations, and TERT promoter mutations.[53]
  - Blistering sunburns and artificial indoor tanning should be avoided to prevent the development of conventional melanomas, which can occur even before adulthood.
  - Lentigo maligna may be seen in patients with xeroderma pigmentosum.[54]
- *CMN-associated melanoma
  - The most common fatal melanomas in young children are CMN associated.
  - CMN-associated melanoma may present within CMN, in other cutaneous locations, or internally (central nervous system or visceral organs). Surgical intervention for multiple or large or giant CMN does not reliably decrease the melanoma risk and is not recommended for malignancy prophylaxis.

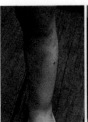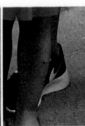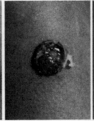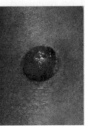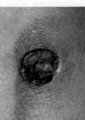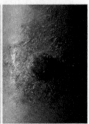

Fig. 4. Evolution of a spitzoid melanoma in a 3-year-old girl before presentation to dermatology, as documented by parent.[46] (*From* Bartenstein DW, Song JS, Nazarian RM, Hawryluk EB. Evolving Childhood Melanoma Monitored by Parental Photodocumentation. J Pediatr. 2017 Jul;186:205–205.e1.)

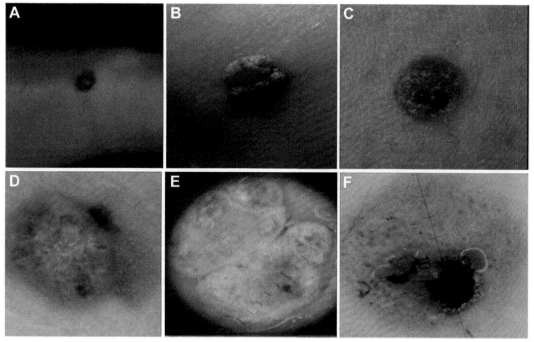

Fig. 5. Pattern 3, pink vascular spitzoid pattern. (*A*) Clinically, hypomelanotic rapid growing tumor on a 14 year old girl. (*B*) Dermoscopy. Polymorphic vascular pattern, with dotted vessels, milky red areas, and the remnants of pigment at the periphery, central shiny white structures. Spitzoid melanoma, Breslow 1.9 mm. (*C*) Clinically, amelanotic pink bump on the lower limb of a 3-year-old girl. (*D*) Dermoscopy. Polymorphic vascular pattern, milky red areas and globules and shiny white structures. Spitzoid melanoma Breslow 5.5 mm. (*E*) Clinically ulcerated amelanotic bump on the lower limb of a 17-year-old girl. (*F*) Dermoscopy. Vascular pattern showing dotted vessels and milky red globules, and ulceration. Spitzoid melanoma, Breslow 1.9 mm. (*From* Carrera C, Scope A, Dusza SW, et al. Clinical and dermoscopic characterization of pediatric and adolescent melanomas: Multicenter study of 52 cases. J Am Acad Dermatol. 2018;78(2):278–288.)

- Melanoma risk increases with CMN size and the presence of multiple lesions.
- All patients with CMN should be taught the importance of inspecting and palpating their birthmarks over the course of their lifetime, and presenting urgently to dermatology with any observed change.
- *Spitz melanoma
  - Spitz melanoma is explored in further detail elsewhere in this article.
  - Spitz melanoma may be amelanotic (pink or red) or pigmented. Malignant tumors often grow rapidly, ulcerate, and bleed.
  - Ancillary genomic testing has yet to be validated in the pediatric population and histopathology remains the gold standard for diagnosis.
  - Fatality from Spitz melanoma has not been reported in a child less than 13 years of age.
- Acral melanoma
  - It can be quite challenging to histologically distinguish benign pediatric acral nevus from acral melanoma. The key features of malignant acral melanoma include pronounced architectural disorder and cytologic abnormalities. Lentiginous melanocytic proliferation and upward migration of melanocytes are nonspecific findings in the pediatric population.[39]
  - The pretest probability of this exceptionally rare entity should be taken into account during evaluation.
- Ocular melanoma
  - Risk factors include oculodermal melanocytosis, choroidal nevi, neurofibromatosis type 1, familial atypical multiple mole and melanoma syndrome, and *BAP1* mutation.[55–57]
  - Ocular melanoma should be considered in the differential diagnosis for children with new ocular symptoms, regardless of risk factors.
- Congenital melanoma
  - Congenital melanoma occurring within the first year of life may occur via transplacental transmission from an affected mother,[58] in association with CMN, or de novo.[59]

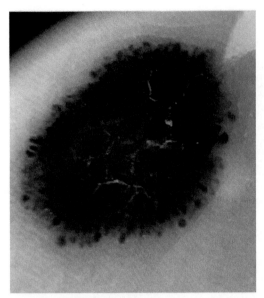

Fig. 6. Pigmented Spitz nevus demonstrating symmetry, lack of ulceration, and characteristic starburst pattern on dermoscopy.

- o Nevi in pregnant women should be evaluated for atypia, malignancy, and sampled promptly if there are any concerning features.[60]
- Melanoma of unknown primary
  - o In general, it is less likely for children to present with malignancies of unknown primary site than adults.[61]

Ancillary Testing

Molecular testing

Molecular tests including but not limited to FISH, comparative genomic hybridization, and PRAME must be interpreted with caution if used for pediatric melanocytic lesions. Despite promising advances in the adult population, studies in pediatrics are limited, as highlighted in the section on spitzoid tumors elsewhere in this article. Molecular studies have neither been validated nor approved in the pediatric population, making results challenging to interpret and use for management decisions.

Sentinel lymph node biopsy

The reliability of SLNB for pediatric melanoma staging is uncertain. Several studies have demonstrated that SLNB positivity is not necessarily indicative of a poor prognosis,[62] but the results are likely confounded by cohorts with young spitzoid melanoma patients. As mentioned elsewhere in this article, a fatality has not been reported in the context of spitzoid melanoma under 13 years of age, and these tumors are likely characterized by a distinct biology. Furthermore, results are likely confounded by cohorts with atypical spitzoid tumors masquerading as spitzoid melanoma. In the past, SLNB was performed to distinguish atypical spitzoid tumors from spitzoid melanomas, but we now know that SLNB does not predict patient survival for patients with atypical spitzoid tumors.

For pediatric patients presenting with nonspitzoid melanomas, it is prudent to recommend SLNB. For very young patients diagnosed with a pediatric spitzoid melanoma, that is unlikely to result in fatality, the decision to pursue SLNB or subsequent treatment is more complex and must be made in careful collaboration with the patient's family and multidisciplinary providers.

CLINICS CARE POINTS

- Pediatric melanoma is exceedingly rare and a high level of suspicion is required for identification. Evolution is likely the most sensitive indicator and close observation can be used for borderline or questionable lesions without acutely concerning features.
- Melanoma presentations and subtypes vary by age group.
- SLNB should be pursued for patients with conventional melanomas, but the decision is complex for prepubertal patients diagnosed with spitzoid melanoma.
- Ancillary genomic testing has not been validated for melanoma diagnosis in the pediatric population.

ACKNOWLEDGEMENTS

Dr E.B. Hawryluk acknowledges the Dermatology Foundation (Pediatric Dermatology Career Development Award) for support.

DISCLOSURE

D.W. Bartenstein: MRK (stock, self); DVA (stock, spouse); ANTM (stock, spouse); PRSC (stock, spouse); AMAG (stock, spouse). E.B. Hawryluk: UpToDate, Inc. (royalty, author/reviewer); Purity Brands, LLC (consultant); Gritstone Oncology, Inc. (salary, stock spouse); PathAI (stock and advisory board, spouse).

REFERENCES

1. Ingordo V, Gentile C, Iannazzone SS, et al. Congenital melanocytic nevus: an epidemiologic study in Italy. Dermatology 2007;214(3):227–30.
2. Stinco G, Argenziano G, Favot F, et al. Absence of clinical and dermoscopic differences between

congenital and noncongenital melanocytic naevi in a cohort of 2-year-old children. Br J Dermatol 2011; 165(6):1303–7.

3. Clemmensen OJ, Kroon S. The histology of "congenital features" in early acquired melanocytic nevi. J Am Acad Dermatol 1988;19(4):742–6.

4. Krengel S. Nevogenesis–new thoughts regarding a classical problem. Am J Dermatopathol 2005; 27(5):456–65.

5. Kinsler VA, Anderson G, Latimer B, et al. Immunohistochemical and ultrastructural features of congenital melanocytic naevus cells support a stem-cell phenotype. Br J Dermatol 2013;169(2): 374–83.

6. Kinsler VA, Thomas AC, Ishida M, et al. Multiple congenital melanocytic nevi and neurocutaneous melanosis are caused by postzygotic mutations in codon 61 of NRAS. J Invest Dermatol 2013;133(9):2229–36.

7. Kinsler V, Shaw AC, Merks JH, et al. The face in congenital melanocytic nevus syndrome. Am J Med Genet A 2012;158a(5):1014–9.

8. Krengel S, Scope A, Dusza SW, et al. New recommendations for the categorization of cutaneous features of congenital melanocytic nevi. J Am Acad Dermatol 2013;68(3):441–51.

9. Vourc'h-Jourdain M, Martin L, Barbarot S. Large congenital melanocytic nevi: therapeutic management and melanoma risk: a systematic review. J Am Acad Dermatol 2013;68(3):493–8.e1-4.

10. Kinsler VA, O'Hare P, Bulstrode N, et al. Melanoma in congenital melanocytic naevi. Br J Dermatol 2017; 176(5):1131–43.

11. Krengel S, Hauschild A, Schafer T. Melanoma risk in congenital melanocytic naevi: a systematic review. Br J Dermatol 2006;155(1):1–8.

12. Kinsler VA, Chong WK, Aylett SE, et al. Complications of congenital melanocytic naevi in children: analysis of 16 years' experience and clinical practice. Br J Dermatol 2008;159(4):907–14.

13. Kim JY, Kim SM, Park KD, et al. A retrospective case series of 10 patients with malignant melanomas arising from small- and medium-sized congenital melanocytic nevi in South Koreans. Indian J Dermatol Venereol Leprol 2021;87(2):293–7.

14. Ott H, Krengel S, Beck O, et al. Multidisciplinary long-term care and modern surgical treatment of congenital melanocytic nevi - recommendations by the CMN surgery network. J Dtsch Dermatol Ges 2019;17(10):1005–16.

15. Kinsler V. Satellite lesions in congenital melanocytic nevi–time for a change of name. Pediatr Dermatol 2011;28(2):212–3.

16. DeDavid M, Orlow SJ, Provost N, et al. Neurocutaneous melanosis: clinical features of large congenital melanocytic nevi in patients with manifest central nervous system melanosis. J Am Acad Dermatol 1996;35(4):529–38.

17. Rhodes AR, Albert LS, Weinstock MA. Congenital nevomelanocytic nevi: proportionate area expansion during infancy and early childhood. J Am Acad Dermatol 1996;34(1):51–62.

18. Yelamos O, Arva NC, Obregon R, et al. A comparative study of proliferative nodules and lethal melanomas in congenital nevi from children. Am J Surg Pathol 2015;39(3):405–15.

19. Waelchli R, Aylett SE, Atherton D, et al. Classification of neurological abnormalities in children with congenital melanocytic naevus syndrome identifies magnetic resonance imaging as the best predictor of clinical outcome. Br J Dermatol 2015;173(3):739–50.

20. Krengel S, Marghoob AA. Current management approaches for congenital melanocytic nevi. Dermatol Clin 2012;30(3):377–87.

21. Charbel C, Fontaine RH, Malouf GG, et al. NRAS mutation is the sole recurrent somatic mutation in large congenital melanocytic nevi. J Invest Dermatol 2014;134(4):1067–74.

22. Gerami P, Paller AS. Making a mountain out of a molehill: NRAS, mosaicism, and large congenital nevi. J Invest Dermatol 2013;133(9):2127–30.

23. Spitz S. Melanomas of childhood. Am J Pathol 1948; 24(3):591–609.

24. Raghavan SS, Peternel S, Mully TW, et al. Spitz melanoma is a distinct subset of spitzoid melanoma. Mod Pathol 2020;33(6):1122–34.

25. Lallas A, Apalla Z, Ioannides D, et al. International Dermoscopy Society. Update on dermoscopy of Spitz/Reed naevi and management guidelines by the International Dermoscopy Society. Br J Dermatol 2017;177(3):645–55.

26. Argenziano G, Agozzino M, Bonifazi E, et al. Natural evolution of Spitz nevi. Dermatology 2011;222(3): 256–60.

27. Hawryluk EB, Duncan LM. The evolving nomenclature of spitzoid proliferations-pediatric outcomes are favorable, regardless of name. Pediatr Dermatol 2020;37(6):1083–4.

28. Tlougan BE, Orlow SJ, Schaffer JV. Spitz nevi: beliefs, behaviors, and experiences of pediatric dermatologists. JAMA Dermatol 2013;149(3):283–91.

29. Davies OMT, Majerowski J, Segura A, et al. A sixteen-year single-center retrospective chart review of Spitz nevi and spitzoid neoplasms in pediatric patients. Pediatr Dermatol 2020;37(6):1073–82.

30. Bartenstein DW, Fisher JM, Stamoulis C, et al. Clinical features and outcomes of spitzoid proliferations in children and adolescents. Br J Dermatol 2019; 181(2):366–72.

31. Gerami P, Scolyer RA, Xu X, et al. Risk assessment for atypical spitzoid melanocytic neoplasms using FISH to identify chromosomal copy number aberrations. Am J Surg Pathol 2013;37(5):676–84.

32. Massi D, Cesinaro AM, Tomasini C, et al. Atypical spitzoid melanocytic tumors: a morphological,

mutational, and FISH analysis. J Am Acad Dermatol 2011;64(5):919–35.

33. Brunetti B, Nino M, Sammarco E, et al. Spitz naevus: a proposal for management. J Eur Acad Dermatol Venereol 2005;19(3):391–3.

34. Lee CY, Sholl LM, Zhang B, et al. Atypical spitzoid neoplasms in childhood: a molecular and outcome study. Am J Dermatopathol 2017;39(3):181–6.

35. Massi D, Tomasini C, Senetta R, et al. Atypical Spitz tumors in patients younger than 18 years. J Am Acad Dermatol 2015;72(1):37–46.

36. Raghavan SS, Wang JY, Kwok S, et al. PRAME expression in melanocytic proliferations with intermediate histopathologic or spitzoid features. J Cutan Pathol 2020;47(12):1123–31.

37. Wiesner T, He J, Yelensky R, et al. Kinase fusions are frequent in Spitz tumours and spitzoid melanomas. Nat Commun 2014;5:3116.

38. Lee S, Barnhill RL, Dummer R, et al. TERT promoter mutations are predictive of aggressive clinical behavior in patients with spitzoid melanocytic neoplasms. Sci Rep 2015;5:11200.

39. Bahrami A, Barnhill RL. Pathology and genomics of pediatric melanoma: A critical reexamination and new insights. Pediatr Blood Cancer 2018;65(2): 10.1002/pbc.26792.

40. Gerami P, Jewell SS, Morrison LE, et al. Fluorescence in situ hybridization (FISH) as an ancillary diagnostic tool in the diagnosis of melanoma. Am J Surg Pathol 2009;33(8):1146–56.

41. Gammon B, Beilfuss B, Guitart J, et al. Enhanced detection of spitzoid melanomas using fluorescence in situ hybridization with 9p21 as an adjunctive probe. Am J Surg Pathol 2012;36(1):81–8.

42. Gerami P, Li G, Pouryazdanparast P, et al. A highly specific and discriminatory FISH assay for distinguishing between benign and malignant melanocytic neoplasms. Am J Surg Pathol 2012;36(6):808–17.

43. Clarke LE, Warf MB, Flake DD 2nd, et al. Clinical validation of a gene expression signature that differentiates benign nevi from malignant melanoma. J Cutan Pathol 2015;42(4):244–52.

44. Hung T, Piris A, Lobo A, et al. Sentinel lymph node metastasis is not predictive of poor outcome in patients with problematic spitzoid melanocytic tumors. Hum Pathol 2013;44(1):87–94.

45. Lallas A, Kyrgidis A, Ferrara G, et al. Atypical Spitz tumours and sentinel lymph node biopsy: a systematic review. Lancet Oncol 2014;15(4):e178–83.

46. Campbell LB, Kreicher KL, Gittleman HR, et al. Melanoma incidence in children and adolescents: decreasing trends in the United States. J Pediatr 2015;166(6):1505–13.

47. Hawryluk EB, Moustafa D, Bartenstein D, et al. A retrospective multicenter study of fatal pediatric melanoma. J Am Acad Dermatol 2020;83(5): 1274–81.

48. Averbook BJ, Lee SJ, Delman KA, et al. Pediatric melanoma: analysis of an international registry. Cancer 2013;119(22):4012–9.

49. Mitkov M, Chrest M, Diehl NN, et al. Pediatric melanomas often mimic benign skin lesions: a retrospective study. J Am Acad Dermatol 2016;75(4):706–11. e704.

50. Bartenstein DW, Song JS, Nazarian RM, Hawryluk EB. Evolving Childhood Melanoma Monitored by Parental Photodocumentation. J Pediatr 2017;186:205–205.e1.

51. Cordoro KM, Gupta D, Frieden IJ, et al. Pediatric melanoma: results of a large cohort study and proposal for modified ABCD detection criteria for children. J Am Acad Dermatol 2013;68(6): 913–25.

52. Carrera C, Scope A, Dusza SW, et al. Clinical and dermoscopic characterization of pediatric and adolescent melanomas: multicenter study of 52 cases. J Am Acad Dermatol 2018;78(2):278–88.

53. Lu C, Zhang J, Nagahawatte P, et al. The genomic landscape of childhood and adolescent melanoma. J Invest Dermatol 2015;135(3):816–23.

54. Barnhill RL, Flotte TJ, Fleischli M, et al. Cutaneous melanoma and atypical Spitz tumors in childhood. Cancer 1995;76(10):1833–45.

55. Vavvas D, Kim I, Lane AM, et al. Posterior uveal melanoma in young patients treated with proton beam therapy. Retina 2010;30(8):1267–71.

56. Al-Jamal RT, Cassoux N, Desjardins L, et al. The pediatric choroidal and ciliary body melanoma study: a survey by the european ophthalmic oncology group. Ophthalmology 2016;123(4):898–907.

57. Soni S, Lee DS, DiVito J Jr, et al. Treatment of pediatric ocular melanoma with high-dose interleukin-2 and thalidomide. J Pediatr Hematol Oncol 2002; 24(6):488–91.

58. Chrysouli K, Tsakanikos M, Stamataki S. A case report of melanoma as acute mastoiditis in a 10-month-old female child. Case Rep Otolaryngol 2019;2019:9641945.

59. Richardson SK, Tannous ZS, Mihm MC Jr. Congenital and infantile melanoma: review of the literature and report of an uncommon variant, pigment-synthesizing melanoma. J Am Acad Dermatol 2002;47(1):77–90.

60. Friedman EB, Scolyer RA, Thompson JF. Management of pigmented skin lesions during pregnancy. Aust J Gen Pract 2019;48(9):621–4.

61. Howman-Giles R, Shaw HM, Scolyer RA, et al. Sentinel lymph node biopsy in pediatric and adolescent cutaneous melanoma patients. Ann Surg Oncol 2010;17(1):138–43.

62. Howman-Giles R, Uren RF, Thompson J. Sentinel lymph node biopsy in pediatric and adolescent patients: a proven technique. Ann Surg 2014;259(6): e86.

An Evidence-Based Approach to Pediatric Melanonychia

Mary E. Lohman, MD[a], Timothy H. McCalmont, MD[b],
Kelly M. Cordoro, MD[c],*

KEYWORDS

- Melanoma • Nevus • Melanonychia • Pediatric • Children • Pigmented lesions

KEY POINTS

In children

- The prevalence of melanonychia varies by age and ethnicity.
- Nail unit melanoma in situ is rare; invasive nail unit melanoma has not been reported.
- Benign causes of melanonychia striata can have a clinical appearance that would be interpreted as potentially malignant in adults: pigmented bands can appear wide; Hutchinson sign and nail dystrophy are common, and lesions may appear atypical dermoscopically and microscopically.
- The threshold to perform a nail unit biopsy for evaluation of melanonychia striata should be higher than that in adult patients; the precise indications for pediatric nail unit biopsy may vary based on individual clinical features and risk factor assessment.
- Expert dermatopathology review is necessary to evaluate pediatric nail unit pigmented lesion biopsies given the atypical features inherent to many benign pediatric nail neoplasms.

INTRODUCTION

Longitudinal melanonychia, or melanonychia striata, represents a pigmented band that runs longitudinally through the nail plate. Although melanonychia striata is less common in children than in adults, it is not rare and is more common in patients with darker skin phenotypes. The underlying causes of melanonychia differ between adults and children. Although most pediatric cases are due to benign nail unit processes, the clinical features may be atypical such that, if present in adult patients, they would be suggestive of malignancy. Furthermore, if biopsied, even benign pigmented lesions of the matrix may have atypical histopathologic characteristics. Thus, the approach to pediatric melanonychia striata, including the decision to biopsy, requires considerations distinct from those in adult patients.

BACKGROUND
Epidemiology

The prevalence of melanonychia striata varies by race and ethnicity. Although melanonychia is common in individuals with dark skin phenotypes, data are limited in some populations. Historically, most data have been reported by ethnicity. The prevalence of melanonychia striata in white individuals is not thought to exceed 1% in adults and children.[1] Although higher rates have been reported in East Asian populations, rates differ significantly within different ethnic groups. Melanonychia striata is less common in adults of Chinese

---

[a] Department of Dermatology, Mayo Clinic, 200 First Street SW, Rochester, MN, 55905, USA; [b] Department of Dermatology and Department of Pathology, University of California, San Francisco, 1701 Divisadero Street, Second Floor, San Francisco, CA 94115; [c] Pediatric Dermatology, Department of Dermatology, University of California, San Francisco, 1701 Divisadero Street, Third Floor, San Francisco, CA 94115, USA
* Corresponding author.
E-mail address: kelly.cordoro@ucsf.edu

Dermatol Clin 40 (2022) 37–49
https://doi.org/10.1016/j.det.2021.09.004

descent (1.3%)[2] compared with Japanese adults (11.4%).[3] Data suggest that rates are higher in Latino individuals with darker skin phototypes; the prevalence among Brazilian adults with skin phototypes IV to VI was found to be 73% with most individuals having multiple affected digits (70% with 2 or more digits affected).[4] A study of black North Americans found pigmented bands of the nails in an average of 77% of individuals older than 20 years.[5]

Overall, the prevalence of melanonychia striata is lower in children. In a large cohort of Chinese patients, melanonychia striata was not seen in those younger than 20 years compared with 0.6% of individuals aged from 20 to 29 years and 1.7% of those more than 50 years old.[2] A similar trend was documented in black North Americans; rates were lower for those younger than 3 years (2.5%) and those aged 3 to 10 years (25%) compared with advanced age groups (up to 96% in individuals more than 50 years old).[5] However, a large study of Japanese individuals showed the opposite trend with a prevalence of 13% in 20-year-olds and no affected individuals older than 60 years.[3] Although pediatric-specific data regarding prevalence of melanonychia striata is limited, it is important to recognize the higher prevalence in children with darker skin phototypes.

Cause

Melanonychia striata is caused by melanin deposition within the nail plate, due to either melanocyte activation (increased melanin production from normally dormant melanocytes in the nail matrix) or a proliferation of melanocytes, frequently referred to as *melanocyte hyperplasia*, in the literature (increased number of nail matrix melanocytes that produce melanin).[6] A strong case can be made that melanocyte hyperplasia is not the best global designation for this group of disorders, but we have used the term in this article in deference to the published record. Most melanocytes of the proximal matrix are quiescent and do not produce melanin, whereas the distal matrix contains a higher number of melanocytes that can be activated to synthesize melanin.[7] When the nail matrix melanocytes are activated, melanin-containing melanosomes are transferred to neighboring cells.[8] As these cells migrate distally and become nail plate corneocytes, a visible pigmented band is formed.

The varying prevalence of melanonychia striata in different skin phototypes is postulated to be a result of variations in melanogenesis. A comparison of nail matrix specimens in white, Japanese, and black adults illustrated a variation in the number and maturity of melanosomes.[8] In nail specimens from white individuals, melanosomes were rare. The melanosomes seen in Japanese and black individuals differed in maturity, with more mature and densely pigmented melanosomes in blacks.

Overall, there are numerous causes of both melanocyte activation and melanocyte hyperplasia of the nail matrix that cause melanonychia (**Table 1**). Melanocyte activation has a broad range of causes, including infection, medications, iatrogenic, primary dermatologic disorders, and systemic disease.[6,9] Both benign and malignant neoplasms can cause an increase in melanocytes.

The common causes of melanonychia striata in adults and children are different (**Table 2**). In adults, melanocyte activation is the most common cause, followed by melanocytic nevi, lentigines, and melanoma, with rates cited in the literature as 73%, 12%, 9%, and 6%, respectively.[10–12] Thus, in adults, nail apparatus melanoma is an important consideration in cases of melanonychia striata. The incidence of melanoma in adults biopsied for melanonychia striata differs between ethnic groups and ranges from 4.3% to 19.8%. Although several studies were small, ungual melanoma was documented in 4.3% of 68 Hispanic patients,[12] 6.2% of 35 Korean patients,[13] 13.5% of 148 French patients,[14] and 19.8% of 96 Iranian patients.[15] However, these studies vary in their methods for selecting patients for biopsy and may overestimate the true incidence of melanoma as a cause of melanonychia striata.

Although melanocyte hyperplasia, and thus melanoma, represents an overall infrequent cause of melanonychia striata in adults, it is estimated that approximately 76% of cases of nail-associated melanoma in adults initially present as melanonychia striata.[16] Rates of nail-associated melanoma as a percentage of overall melanomas also differ by ethnicity, with higher rates in patients with skin of color. In white patients, nail-associated melanoma represents only 0.2% to 3.4% of all melanomas.[16,17] However, nail-associated melanomas are reported to represent 23% of all melanomas in Japanese patients and 25% of all melanomas in black patients.[11]

In pediatric patients, melanocyte hyperplasia is the most common cause of melanonychia striata. Nevi are the most common cause of longitudinal melanonychia, estimated at between 48% and 94%,[11,18,19] with varying rates attributed to ethnic differences. Lentigines are thought to be the second most common cause of melanonychia striata in children, accounting for 30% to 67% of cases.[19,20] Although there is no official reported rate for melanocyte activation, it is likely the third

Table 1
Common[a] causes of melanonychia

Causes of Melanonychia/Melanonychia Striata (Single or Multiple Digits)[6,9]	
Melanocyte Activation	**Melanocyte Proliferation**
Congenital • Alkaptonuria • Peutz-Jeghers • Laugier-Hunziker Infectious • Onychomycosis • Paronychia • Verruca vulgaris Inflammatory • Primary dermatologic disorders (lichen planus, lichen striatus, psoriasis) • Graft-versus-host disease Iatrogenic • Ingestions (arsenic, mercury, thallium) • Trauma (especially sports) • Radiation • Phototherapy Idiopathic/physiologic • Ethnic melanonychia • Pregnancy Medications • Antibacterial (sulfonamides, tetracyclines) • Antifungal (ketoconazole, fluconazole, voriconazole) • Antimalarials • Chemotherapies (bleomycin, busulfan, cyclophosphamide, doxorubicin, 5-fluorouracil, hydroxyurea, methotrexate) • Others (amlodipine, ibuprofen, steroids, phenytoin, zidovudine) Metabolic/endocrine disorders • Addison disease • Cushing syndrome • Thyrotoxicosis • Hemochromatosis • Porphyria Neoplastic • Pigmented squamous cell carcinoma in situ • Basal cell carcinoma • Mucous cyst	Benign • Congenital melanocytic nevus • Acquired melanocytic nevus • Lentigo Malignant • Melanoma in situ • Invasive melanoma

[a] The list is not exhaustive; other rare causes may exist.

Table 2
Common causes of melanonychia/melanonychia striata in adult versus pediatric populations ranked by incidence reported in the literature

Common Causes of Melanonychia/Melanonychia Striata Ranked by Age Group	
Adult Patients	**Pediatric Patients**
1. Melanocyte activation: 73%[10]	1. Nevi: 48%–94%[11,18,19]
2. Nevi: 12%[11]	2. Lentigo: 30%–67%[19,20]
3. Lentigo: 9%[11]	3. Melanocyte activation
4. Melanoma: 6%[12]	4. Melanoma: rare

most common cause of melanonychia in children and likely a more common cause of melanonychia in the setting of skin of color. Finally, pediatric melanoma as a cause of melanonychia is rare, with few case reports in the literature.

Notably, there are no documented cases of pediatric invasive melanoma presenting as melanonychia striata. In the 3 reported cases of invasive ungual melanoma in pediatrics, 1 presented with a painful subungual nodule[21] and 2 cases presented as changing pigmented lesions of the nail fold or periungual skin.[22,23] However, invasive ungual melanoma initially presenting as melanonychia striata in childhood has been postulated. In one case report, a 19-year-old noted a 2-year history of nail thickening and growth of longstanding melanonychia striata. At the time of biopsy, invasive melanoma was diagnosed, thus the investigators note that this could represent the first case of pediatric invasive melanoma presenting with melanonychia striata.[18]

When compared with invasive melanoma, pediatric melanoma in situ (MIS) presenting as longitudinal melanonychia has been documented in multiple case reports. There are 15 case reports in the English language literature,[24–32] but the diagnoses of some cases are called into question with the description of pediatric subungual atypical melanocytic hyperplasia (AMH). Recently, Cooper and colleagues[20] used AMH to describe pediatric nail unit neoplasm with increased single melanocytes with suprabasalar and pagetoid spread. The investigators note that the histopathologic characteristics of these lesions, including variable nuclear atypia, are similar to the described findings in prior case reports interpreted as pediatric ungual MIS. The information regarding each previously reported case of pediatric nail unit MIS is inherently limited given the presentation by case report with limited photomicrographs. Thus, confirmation or validation of the original diagnosis of MIS is challenging.

Challenges in Diagnosis

The histology of the nail unit is unique. The nail matrix and the resident melanocytes are distinct in 3 ways: (1) nail matrix melanocytes are typically quiescent, (2) melanocytes are less numerous in the nail matrix compared with the epidermis, and (3) melanocytes are commonly located in the suprabasilar layer of the nail matrix.[33] Thus, it is common to see suprabasilar melanocytes within the nail matrix,[7,34] which may be misconstrued as an indication of melanoma when interpreting clinically concerning cases of melanonychia striata.

Examination of pediatric pigmented nail lesions presents additional challenges. In general, specimens are small and benign pediatric nail neoplasms can have atypical histopathologic features.[35] Pediatric nail unit nevi and lentigines have features commonly associated with MIS, such as nuclear enlargement and pagetoid spread.[34,35] Furthermore, multinucleated giant cells, high melanocyte density, and confluence of single melanocytes are not uncommon.[36] Multinucleated cells are often an indicator of malignant neoplasms in adults, whereas multinucleation can be seen in benign causes of melanonychia striata in young patients.[36]

Diagnosis of pediatric nail unit melanoma is further complicated by the lack of absolute criteria for early nail-associated melanoma.[17] The rarity of pediatric nail unit melanomas also dictates that few dermatopathologists have expertise in this area.[35] Changes in early subungual MIS are subtle and challenging to identify.[25] One of the earliest microscopic changes is an increase in the density of intraepidermal melanocytes.[34] In addition, nuclear atypicality and pagetoid spread can be focal in early melanoma.[37] The subtlety inherent to this diagnosis has led to the recent exploration of additional histopathologic testing to validate the diagnosis in this context.

The options for external validation of a diagnosis of nail unit melanoma are limited. Immunostains such as S100, Melan-A, and HMB-45 simply define the distribution of melanocytes and may highlight architectural disorder; however, they do not distinguish between benign and malignant melanocytes. Recently, fluorescence in situ hybridization (FISH), P16 staining, and Ki 67 proliferation rates have been used to help support the diagnosis of pediatric nail MIS in case reports.[24,25,29] However, robust data in pediatrics are limited.

FISH has been used with a high sensitivity and specificity for diagnosing melanoma in general, reported as 94% and 98%, respectively.[38] However, FISH has only recently been applied to nail matrix melanomas. Data in adults suggest that nail-associated melanomas show similar abnormalities to acral melanomas, including gain of RREB1 (Ras-responsive element-binding protein 1), CCND1 (cyclin D1), and MYC and loss of MYB.[39] Compared with melanomas at other locations, loss of CDKN2A (cyclin-dependent kinase inhibitor 2A) seems to be less common in nail-associated melanoma, whereas gain of CCND1 is less common in melanomas of other sites.[39] Data in pediatrics are limited; when FISH was applied to 3 nail neoplasms concerning for MIS, gain of CCND1 was only identified in 1 of 3 cases.[25] No copy number aberrations in CCND1 were identified in 13 cases of pediatric nail unit nevi and lentigines.[36] Although FISH may aid in risk stratification of some lesions by identifying previously documented genomic aberrations observed in adult tumors, the lack of data regarding other potential gains and losses in pediatric nail unit melanoma is limiting.

Both loss of P16 and elevated Ki 67 proliferation rates have been used, generally, to diagnose pediatric melanoma, but meaningful data for nail tumors are lacking. In pediatrics, loss of P16 has been useful to distinguish melanoma from conventional melanocytic nevi and Spitz nevi.[40] While recognizing that P16 staining has not been used extensively in pediatric nail matrix neoplasms, one recent case report used loss of P16 to support their diagnosis of pediatric nail matrix MIS.[29] Similarly, high Ki 67 proliferation rates have been used adjunctively to distinguish between benign and malignant neoplasms in pediatrics, including differentiating Spitz nevi and melanoma. A high Ki 67 proliferation rate was used in a recent case report to support a diagnosis of pediatric nail matrix MIS.[24] Despite its promises, it is important to note that Ki 67 is challenging to interpret in minimally nested proliferations. Thus, its use in pigmented pediatric nail neoplasms, which classically lack extensive nesting, may be limited.

Although not yet applied to pediatric cases, PRAME (preferentially expressed antigen in melanoma) may be a promising future adjunct immunostain. PRAME is highly expressed in most melanoma subtypes, including in more than 94% of acral melanomas.[41] Currently there are no published data on PRAME expression specifically in nail matrix nevi or nail unit melanomas. However, based on high expression in adult acral melanomas, it seems likely that PRAME expression can be a valuable diagnostic tool.

EVALUATION

The atypical clinical features of pediatric melanonychia striata are well documented and necessitate a unique approach compared with the recommended approach to melanonychia striata in adults. Clinical features typically considered concerning for malignancy in adults are commonly seen in benign cases of pediatric melanonychia striata including broad bandwidth, nail dystrophy, Hutchinson sign, and clinical change.

Atypical Clinical Features

Case series highlight that even among cases with concerning clinical features, pediatric nail MIS is rare. **Table 3** summarizes 11 case series of melanonychia and its histopathology performed at 8

different universities, as well as several additional international hospitals and outpatient clinics.[10,15,16,18–20,25,36,42–44] Overall, only 2 cases of MIS were identified of 208 cases.[25] One case in a black 4-year-old male showed a black 6-mm changing pigmented band of the left second finger with no Hutchinson sign. The second case in a 6-year-old male showed a brown 6-mm changing pigmented band of the left great toe. Two additional cases were identified as atypical junctional melanocytic hyperplasia in this case series concerning for MIS. FISH was performed on both lesions with a rendered diagnosis of MIS, one of which showed a copy number aberration supporting the initial diagnosis of MIS, whereas the other failed to show any abnormalities. The investigators noted that this negative result does not exclude the diagnosis of MIS given the possibility of other genetic abnormalities outside of the probed loci.[25] Over the past 10 years at our center, we have biopsied 10 nail matrices in pediatric patients with clinically worrisome melanonychia. All cases were benign (see **Table 3**).

Overall, the data from the literature as well as our own clinical experience highlight the atypical clinical features of pediatric melanonychia striata including wide pigment bands, nail dystrophy, Hutchinson sign, and progressive clinical change (**Fig. 1**). Given the frequency of atypical clinical features of pediatric melanonychia combined with the infrequency of pediatric nail matrix melanoma, the ability to risk stratify patients is a challenge. Some investigators have concluded that the most promising feature suggesting a diagnosis of nail matrix melanoma may be an *older age of onset*.[18]

Melanonychia striata is commonly wider in children compared with adults. Although 3 mm has previously been used as a threshold to identify concerning lesions, this is unlikely to be a helpful measure in pediatric patients. Pediatric pigmented bands are wider than seen in adults, sometimes up to 3 times wider. In one study, melanonychia was 3.5 times wider among Asian children compared with adults.[45] When pooling data from available case series (see **Table 3**), 50% of biopsied cases of pediatric melanonychia striata were more than 3 mm or were wider than 50% of the nail plate. It has been suggested that a more accurate measure may be grouping the width of pigmentation into 3 groups by nail involvement: less than one-third of the nail plate involved, between one-third and two-thirds, and more than two-thirds of the width of the nail plate. Most subungual melanomas involve more than two-thirds of the nail plate.[46] However, this has not been validated in pediatric patients.

Nail dystrophy is also common in pediatric melanonychia striata. Some studies do not report

Table 3
Summary of available case series of pediatric melanonychia striata

Location	Cases	Skin of Color	Melanoma cases	>3 mm or >50% nail	Hutchinson	Pseudo-Hutchinson	Dystrophy	Multi colored	Evolving
Pellegrin Hospital, France[43]	5	NR	0	2	NR	NR	NR	NR	NR
Bologna & Cannes Nail Center[10]	11	NR	0	7	2	NR	2	2	2
International outpatient clinic[19]	40	18% phototype IV+	0	12	9	NR	NR	12	NR
Northwestern University[20]	30	NR	0	13	4	4	2	7	10
Tehran University[15]	9	All Iranian	0	NR	NR	NR	NR	NR	NR
Hallym University, Korea[44]	21	All phototype III	0	16	5	NR	4	3	NR
National Taiwan University[18]	18	NR	0	12	14	2	3	8	17
Harvard & University of Michigan[25]	11	55% nonwhite	2 (MIS)	6	5	NR	NR	NR	10
2 outpatient clinics, Singapore[42]	14	All Asian descent	0	2	2	NR	NR	NR	12
Fundan University, Shanghai[36]	35	All Chinese	0	22	14	9	5	NR	NR
University Gdansk, Poland[16]	4	50% phototype III+	0	4	1	2	0	4	1
University of California, San Francisco[a]	10		0	8	2	1	2	5	10
Total cases	**208**		**2**	**104**	**58**	**17**	**18**	**41**	**62**
Percent of total cases (198)			**1%**	**50%**	**28%**	**9%**	**9%**	**20%**	**30%**

Each case series represents a pooled summary of institutional cases of pediatric melanonychia striata with available histopathology. Thus, only biopsied cases of pediatric melanonychia are reflected. All available patient and clinical characteristics reported in case series are summarized, with missing data indicated.
Abbreviation: NR, not reported.
[a] Unpublished data.

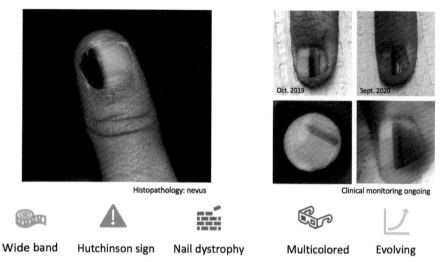

Fig. 1. Common features of pediatric melanonychia/melanonychia striata exemplified by 2 cases. These features are considered atypical when seen in melanonychia striata in adults; however, data show that these features are common in cases of pediatric melanonychia striata.

dystrophy, whereas pooled data from case series suggest that 9% of pediatric melanonychia is associated with nail dystrophy and none of these cases showed underlying MIS (see **Table 3**). In a study of pediatric nail matrix nevi alone, rates of nail dystrophy were as high as 60% (12 of 20) and were associated with wider pigmented bands.[45] The investigators postulate that nail dystrophy in pediatric nail unit nevi may have a mechanism similar to large pediatric congenital nevi, which are often associated with alterations in surrounding skin structures such as hypertrichosis or appendageal hypotrophy.[45] Others have attributed nail dystrophy to softening of the nail plate as melanin is incorporated into the plate's sulfur and keratin proteins.[47]

The Hutchinson sign, or extension of pigment onto periungual tissue, has historically been considered pathognomonic for nail-associated melanoma, because it is associated with the radial growth phase of subungual melanoma.[48] However, the hallmark status of the Hutchinson sign has been challenged given numerous mimicking conditions that can present with subungual and periungual pigmentation. These conditions include nail unit nevi and many of the causes of melanocyte activation including ethnic melanonychia, nonmelanoma skin cancer of the nail unit, infections, medications, trauma, and systemic causes of melanocyte activation (pregnancy, Addison disease).[49,50] "Pseudo-Hutchinson" sign has been used to refer to these banal causes of periungual pigmentation, whereas both "pseudo-Hutchinson" and "false Hutchinson" have been used to refer to the illusion of pigment within the epidermis due to transparency of periungual tissue.[49] Pooled data again suggest that both

the Hutchinson and pseudo-Hutchinson signs are common in pediatric melanonychia striata, present in 37% of cases (see **Table 3**). Some have attributed the high prevalence of the pseudo-Hutchinson, or false Hutchinson, sign in pediatrics to the darker nature of nail matrix nevi in kids.[47] In addition to visibility of pigment through the proximal nail fold, pigment emanating from matrix nevi has also been observed in the lateral nail folds and hyponychium.[45]

Both progression and regression have been documented in benign pediatric nail matrix neoplasms. Although not reported in all studies, pooled data suggest that more than 30% of pediatric melanonychia striata cases were evolving at the time of biopsy yet still show benign causes (see **Table 3**). However, some institutions and practitioners use clinical change as a threshold for biopsy, so these data may overestimate the prevalence of change in pediatrics. One study showed high rates of narrowing or disappearance (up to 76%) in a series of adult and pediatric nail matrix nevi.[45] Proposed mechanisms of narrowing pigment bands include the decrease of melanin production with persistence of the nevus as well as apoptosis of nevus cells.[44,51] Thus, the most compelling feature suggesting malignancy in general—evolution or progressive change—is relatively common in benign cases of pediatric melanonychia striata.

Atypical Dermatoscopic Features

Numerous dermatoscopic findings of nail unit nevi have been explored as predictors of melanoma. In addition to wide pigment bands, nail plate dystrophy, and Hutchinson sign, dermatoscopic documentation of pigment variegation, granular pigment, or gray and black coloration have been highlighted as clues to ungual melanoma in adults.[52] Of note, melanocyte activation in skin phototypes IV to VI also demonstrates high rates of irregularly pigmented lines on dermoscopy (76%) as well as dark brown or black pigmented backgrounds (71% and 29%, respectively).[4]

Dermatoscopic findings of pediatric melanonychia striata are different from those of adults. When evaluating the dermatoscopic features of nail nevi in kids, one study documented a higher prevalence of atypical features including dark and multicolored bands, pseudo-Hutchinson sign, triangle sign, and pigment dots and globules.[47] Overall, irregularly colored bands in pediatric nail matrix nevi are widely accepted; consensus guidelines on dermatoscopic features predictive of nail unit melanoma from the International Study Group on Melanonychia highlight the importance of irregularly colored brown bands and dark background pigment, but it should be noted that width and spacing of bands do not indicate melanoma in kids.[53] In addition, whereas the triangle sign has been estimated to be an indicator of nail melanoma in 5% to 25% of white patients, 25% of pediatric nail nevi according to one study demonstrate the same finding.[47]

DISCUSSION

Although pediatric melanonychia striata can have many causes, it is most commonly due to benign nail matrix nevi or lentigines. The atypical histopathologic features of pediatric nail matrix lentigines and nevi make the microscopic distinction between benign and malignant nail matrix neoplasms challenging. FISH, P16, and PRAME do provide potential opportunities for supporting a diagnosis of MIS in pediatric melanonychia striata, but their use in the literature and in practice is limited. Without validated criteria or an external histopathologic marker for diagnosis, it is possible that pediatric nail unit melanoma may be overcalled. Therefore, it is critical that biopsy specimens are reviewed by dermatopathologists with experience and expertise in pediatric pigmented nail lesions. Some pathologists may overcall because the implications of missing the diagnosis are high. However, the implications of overdiagnosis can be morbid. In the past, treatment favored excision of the entire nail apparatus, or in invasive cases, amputation of the distal phalanx. Now, conservative re-excision or Mohs surgery is considered for MIS and conservative re-excision is also considered for thin melanomas. However,

comparative studies and pediatric data are lacking.

In adults, many predictive models have been proposed to help early identification of high-risk nail lesions. The "ABCDEF rule" was developed to help early clinical identification of subungual melanoma.[54] These criteria cover features such as age (50–70 year old), breadth 3 mm or larger, clinical change, digit involved (thumb or hallux), extension of pigment to periungual tissue (Hutchinson sign), and family (or personal) history of melanoma. Although this is widely cited in the literature, a subsequent study attempting to use it in clinical practice for adults found that only a wide pigment band was associated with ungual melanoma.[55] Another group subsequently proposed the ABCD rule for subungual MIS using the following criteria: age greater than 18 years, brown bands in a brown background on dermoscopy, color in periungual skin (Hutchinson sign), and pigment restricted to one digit.[56] Although a high sensitivity and specificity were reported in a mixed group of pediatric and adult patients (100% and 96.6%, respectively),[56] sensitivity and specificity for pediatric patients alone is lacking.

Similarly, predictive models using dermatoscopic features have been proposed to identify ungual MIS. One recent study found a statistically significant association of several dermoscopic findings including asymmetry, border fading, multicolor bands, width greater than 3 mm or greater than 6 mm, and presence of Hutchinson.[57] Although this predictive scoring model demonstrated reliable diagnostic value (reported sensitivity of 89% and specificity of 62%), it has not been validated in pediatric patients.

The lack of clinical models for evaluation and management of pediatric melanonychia striata is a reflection of its inherent atypical clinical and dermatoscopic features. Therefore, within the literature, there are varying recommendations regarding the threshold to perform a biopsy. Most advocate a conservative approach to biopsy, which favors clinical monitoring, often in conjunction with photography and dermoscopy.[9,20,44] Rapid growth is the one clinical feature that many identify as a threshold for biopsy.[19,43]

Recommendations

The approach to melanonychia and consideration of nail matrix biopsies in the pediatric population requires careful consideration of multiple factors in addition to the appearance and history of the nail lesion: individual risk factors (strong family history of melanoma; history of radiation or immunosuppression), level of family concern and preferences, and the need in younger patients for general anesthesia to perform the procedure. Similar to others in the field who have proposed an algorithmic approach,[58] our institutional experience with pediatric melanonychia combined with existing data has led to a principled approach that favors clinical monitoring in most cases and shared decision making with caregivers in all cases (**Fig. 2**).

First, a detailed clinical history is important. An inventory of the lesional history—onset, course, associated symptoms, extrinsic factors such as trauma from sports or activities, past medical history, medications, family history, and social history—is imperative to put the examination findings in context and attempt to risk stratify. In

the case of melanonychia affecting multiple nails, a thorough history will help to identify many potential causes of melanonychia including ethnic melanonychia, idiopathic melanocyte activation from repetitive trauma due to sports, medical conditions, and medications. Notably, within the extensive list of causes of melanocyte activation (see **Table 1**), we have frequently observed trauma as a cause of melanonychia striata, especially in skin of color. For single nail melanonychia, a history documenting onset, rate of change, and history of trauma is important to guide decision making.

Next, a thorough examination of all nails and ideally the skin and hair should be performed. We recommend a baseline examination that

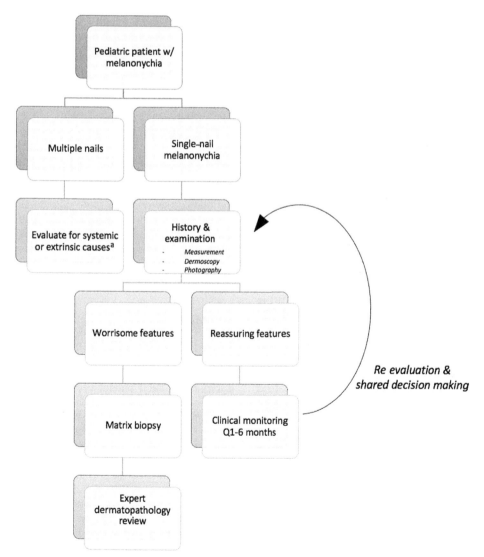

Fig. 2. Proposed clinical approach to pediatric melanonychia striata/longitudinal melanonychia. See section Recommendations for full discussion regarding proposed approach. Q, every; w/, with. [a] See **Table 1**.

includes measurement of the width of the proximal and distal aspect of the bands, lateral bandwidth, presence of pigment in the nail folds (true pigment or apparent pigment), presence of nail dystrophy and anatomic distortion of any aspect of the nail unit, and a dermatoscopic evaluation. Clinical and dermatoscopic (if possible) photographs should be obtained to document change over time. Given the availability of high-quality photography through personal smartphones, we also advocate for photographs to be taken with a patient's personal device to facilitate self-monitoring.

For single nail melanonychia, timing of follow-up for monitoring depends on the clinical scenario and should be individualized. Closer interval of follow-up initially (1–3 months) with reduced frequency over time (3–6 months) in cases of stability is a reasonable approach. All follow-up visits should include interval history and examination with repeat measurements, dermoscopy, comparison with old photographs, and new photographs for serial monitoring.

Decision making for lesions with worrisome clinical features, rapid change, or occurring in high-risk patients is nuanced and also individualized. Given that clinical change can be a common finding in benign causes of pediatric melanonychia striata and may be due to natural growth of a nevus, determining what *significant change* is for an individual patient is the challenge. Rapid growth over the course of weeks to a few months, with or without nail dystrophy, periungual pigmentation, and other clinical changes should prompt a discussion with family and consideration of a biopsy. In the presence of significant clinical change as defined for and identified in an individual patient, we recommend either close-interval or serial reevaluation of the clinical scenario to determine if a biopsy is necessary.

Discussion with family about the risks and benefits of observation versus biopsy is important. The conversation should acknowledge the low prevalence of nail unit melanoma in pediatrics and the atypical clinical features of benign neoplasms such as nevi and lentigines. Shared decision making with caregivers is critical, and offering a medical opinion about the lesion helps to frame the discussion. If, on balance, the clinical context (lesional and patient characteristics), risk factors, family preferences. and circumstances warrant histopathologic investigation, then one should proceed with a biopsy.

As discussed in detail, available data and our combined clinical experience do not clearly delineate a consistent set of criteria for which an immediate matrix biopsy is mandatory in pediatric patients. However, some clinical features are more compelling, and a biopsy is recommended for cases featuring rapid growth out of proportion to what would be expected for benign nevus evolution, presence of a subungual mass, extensive nail unit anatomic changes, extensive and progressive spread of periungual pigmentation, and symptoms such as nontraumatic bleeding or pain. Ideally, the physician performing the biopsy will have had training and experience in pediatric nail surgery, because there are multiple ways to perform nail matrix biopsies with specific indications for each.[59,60] Finally, expert dermatopathology review is a must. Given the nuances inherent to the diagnosis of benign versus malignant pediatric nail matrix lesions and the stakes of overcalling or undercalling, the importance of review by an experienced dermatopathologist and ideally a collaborative approach to a consensus diagnosis cannot be overemphasized.

LIMITATIONS

One of the limitations in this work is the lack of existing data further stratifying pediatric patient age and risk. It is possible that, similar to cutaneous melanoma in pediatric patients, age makes a difference in presentation and natural history.[61] In young children, congenital or acquired nevi of the matrix may undergo more change as part of natural evolution and maturation, whereas in older children and adolescents, similar changes may be more suggestive of the presence or potential for malignant degeneration. More data are needed to fully assess age as a risk factor.

SUMMARY

Based on available data, we offer a clinical approach to management of pediatric melanonychia striata. We recommend an individualized approach to each patient consisting of comprehensive evaluation, serial reassessment, and involvement of caregivers in decisions to observe versus biopsy. Given the challenges related to interpretation of biopsies obtained from the nail unit, biopsy specimens of pigmented lesions should be reviewed by dermatopathologists with experience in pediatric nail matrix neoplasms. These recommendations are not formal guidelines and will not be relevant in all situations. Medical decision making as it relates to pediatric melanonychia requires careful assessment, frequent reassessment, and consideration of the unique circumstances of each individual patient.

CLINICS CARE POINTS

- Nail matrix nevi are the most common cause of pediatric melanonychia striata and can present with irregular, wide pigment bands and associated nail dystrophy and Hutchinson sign.

- Malignant causes of pediatric melanonychia striata are rare; only MIS has been reported.

- FISH and P16 may be useful adjuncts in distinguishing between benign and malignant causes of pediatric melanonychia striata, but all dermatopathology review should be executed by dermatopathologists experienced with pediatric nail matrix neoplasms.

- Expert consensus favors clinical monitoring of pediatric melanonychia striata; biopsy should be pursued in cases of significant clinical change or severely atypical features in individualized patients.

DISCLOSURE

The authors have nothing to disclose.

REFERENCES

1. Kopf A, Waldot E. Melanonychia striata*. Australas J Dermatol 1980;21(59):59–70.
2. Leung AKC, Robson WLM, Liu EKH, et al. Melanonychia striata in Chinese children and adults. Int J Dermatol 2007;46(9):920–2.
3. Kawamura T, Nishihara K, Kawasakiya S. Pigmentatio longitudinalis striata unguium and the pigmentation of nail plate in Addison disease. Jpn J Dermatol 1958;68:76–88.
4. Astur MDMM, Farkas CB, Junqueira JP, et al. Reassessing melanonychia striata in phototypes IV, V, and VI patients. Dermatol Surg 2016;42(2):183–90.
5. Leyden JJ, Spott DA, Goldschmidt H. Diffuse and banded melanin pigmentation in nails. Arch Dermatol 1972;105(4):548–50.
6. Baran R, Kechijian P. Longitudinal melanonychia (melanonychia striata): Diagnosis and management. J Am Acad Dermatol 1989;21(6):1165–75.
7. Perrin C, Michiels JF, Pisani A, et al. Anatomic distribution of melanocytes in normal nail unit: an immunohistochemical investigation. Am J Dermatopathol 1997;19(5):462–7.
8. Hashimoto K. Ultrastructure of the human toenail. I. Proximal nail matrix. J Invest Dermatol 1971;56(3):235–46.
9. Leung AKC, Lam JM, Leong KF, et al. Melanonychia striata: clarifying behind the Black Curtain. A review on clinical evaluation and management of the 21st century. Int J Dermatol 2019;58(11):1239–45.
10. Tosti A, Baran R, Piraccini M, et al. Nail matrix nevi : a clinical and histopathologic study of twenty-two patients. J Am Acad Dermatol 1996;34(5):765–71.
11. André J, Lateur N. Pigmented nail disorders. Dermatol Clin 2006;24(3):329–39.
12. Dominguez-Cherit J, Roldan-Marin R, Pichardo-Velazquez P, et al. Melanonychia, melanocytic hyperplasia, and nail melanoma in a Hispanic population. J Am Acad Dermatol 2008;59(5):785–91.
13. Jin H, Kim JM, Kim GW, et al. Diagnostic criteria for and clinical review of melanonychia in Korean patients. J Am Acad Dermatol 2016;74(6):1121–7.
14. Ronger S, Touzet S, Ligeron C, et al. Dermoscopic examination of nail pigmentation. Arch Dermatol 2002;138(10):1327–33.
15. Kamyab K, Abdollahi M, Nezam-Eslami E, et al. Longitudinal melanonychia in an Iranian population: a study of 96 patients. Int J Women's Dermatol 2016; 2(2):49–52.
16. Sobjanek M, Sławińska M, Romaszkiewicz A, et al. Childhood longitudinal melanonychia: case series from Poland. Postep Dermatol Alergol 2020;37(2): 195–201.
17. Thai K, Young R, Sinclair RD. Nail apparatus melanoma CME 2001. p. 1–13. Available at: papers2:// publication/uuid/16D3A62B-692E-40F1-B6C9-D250 CF5159A6%20.
18. Tseng Y-T, Liang C, Liau J-Y, et al. Longitudinal melanonychia: Differences in etiology are associated with patient age at diagnosis. Dermatology 2017; 233:446–55.
19. Goettmann-Bonvallot S, Andre J, Belaich S. Longitudinal melanonychia in children: a clinical and histopathologic study of 40 cases. J Am Acad Dermatol 1999;41(1):17–22.
20. Cooper C, Arva NC, Lee C, et al. A clinical, histopathologic, and outcome study of melanonychia striata in childhood. J Am Acad Dermatol 2015; 72(5):773–9.
21. Takata M, Maruo K, Kageshita T, et al. Two cases of unusual acral melanocytic tumors: illustration of molecular cytogenetics as a diagnostic tool. Hum Pathol 2003;34(1):89–92.
22. Lyall D. Malignant melanoma in infancy. JAMA 1967; 202:1153.
23. Uchiyama M, Minemura K. Two cases of malignant melanoma in young persons. Nippon Hifuka Gakkai Zasshi 1979;89:668.
24. Akay BN, Kirmizi A, Bostanci S, et al. Paediatric melanoma of the nail unit with rapid progression: a case report with dermatoscopic follow-up and intraoperative dermatoscopic images. Australas J Dermatol 2020;61(1):46–8.

25. Khatri SS, Wang M, Harms KL, et al. Subungual atypical lentiginous melanocytic proliferations in children and adolescents: a clinicopathologic study. J Am Acad Dermatol 2018;79(2):327–36.e2.

26. Motta A, Lopez C, Acosta A, et al. Subungual melanoma in situ in a hispanic girl treated with functional resection and reconstruction with onychocutaneous toe free flap. Arch Derm 2007;143(12):1600–2.

27. Kiryu H. Malignant melanoma In situ arising in the nail unit of a child. J Dermatol 1998;25(1):41–4.

28. Kato T, Usuba Y, Takematsu H, et al. A rapidly growing pigmented nail streak resulting in diffuse melanosis. Cancer 1989;64:1989.

29. Bonamonte, Arpaia. In situ melanoma of the nail unit presenting as a rapid growing longitudinal melanonychia in a 9-year-old white boy. Dermatol Surg 2014;40(10):1154–7.

30. Antonovich DD, Grin C, Grant-Kels JM. Childhood subungual melanoma in situ in diffuse nail melanosis beginning as expanding longitudinal melanonychia. Pediatr Dermatol 2005;22(3):210–2.

31. Tosti A, Piraccini B, Cagalli A, et al. In situ melanoma of the nail unit in children : report of two cases in fair-skinned Caucasian children. Pediatr Dermatol 2012; 29(1):79–83.

32. Iorizzo M, Tosti A, Chiacchio N Di, et al. Nail melanoma in children: differential diagnosis and management. Dermatol Surg 2008;34(7):974–8.

33. Higashi N. Melanocytes of nail matrix and nail pigmentation. Arch Dermatol 1968;97(5):570–4.

34. Amin B, Nehal KS, Jungbluth AA, et al. Histologic distinction between subungual Lentigo and Melanoma. Am J Surg Pathol 2008;32(6):835–43.

35. Theunis A, Richert B, Sass U, et al. Immunohistochemical study of 40 cases of longitudinal melanonychia. Am J Dermatopathol 2011;33(1):27–34.

36. Ren J, Ren M, Kong YY, et al. Clinicopathological diversity and outcome of longitudinal melanonychia in children and adolescents: analysis of 35 cases identified by excision specimens. Histopathology 2020; 77(3):380–90.

37. Izumi M, Ohara K, Hoashi T, et al. Subungual melanoma: histological examination of 50 cases from early stage to bone invasion. J Dermatol 2008; 35(11):695–703.

38. Gerami P, Li G, Pouryazdanparast P, et al. A highly specific and discriminatory fish assay for distinguishing between benign and malignant melanocytic neoplasms. Am J Surg Pathol 2012;36(6):808–17.

39. Romano RC, Shon W, Sukov WR. Malignant melanoma of the nail apparatus: a fluorescence in situ hybridization analysis of 7 cases. Int J Surg Pathol 2016;24(6):512–8.

40. Al Dhaybi R, Agoumi M, Gagné I, et al. P16 expression: a marker of differentiation between childhood malignant melanomas and Spitz nevi. J Am Acad Dermatol 2011;65(2):357–63.

41. Lezcano C, Jungbluth AA, Nehal KS, et al. PRAME expression in melanocytic tumors. Am J Surg Pathol 2018;42(11):1456–65.

42. Tan W, Mbbs T, Yuan D, et al. Should we biopsy melanonychia striata in Asian children ? A retrospective observational study. Pediatr Dermatol 2019;36:864–8.

43. Leaute-Labreze C, Bioulac-Sage P, Taieb A. Longitudinal melanonychia in Children: a study of 8 cases. Arch Derm 1996;132:167–9.

44. Lee MK, Seo SB, Jung JY, et al. Longitudinal melanonychia in childhood: a clinical and histopathological review of Korean patients. Eur J Dermatol 2017; 27(3):275–80.

45. Lee JH, Lim Y, Park J, et al. Clinicopathologic features of 28 cases of nail matrix nevi (NMNs) in Asians: comparison between children and adults. J Am Dermatol 2017;78(3):479–89.

46. Benati E, Ribero S, Longo C, et al. Clinical and dermoscopic clues to differentiate pigmented nail bands: an International Dermoscopy Society study. J Eur Acad Dermatol Venereol 2017;31(4):732–6.

47. Ohn J, Choe YS, Mun JH. Dermoscopic features of nail matrix nevus (NMN) in adults and children: a comparative analysis. J Am Acad Dermatol 2016; 75(3):535–40.

48. Patterson RH, Helwig EB. Subungual malignant melanoma: a clinical-pathologic study. Cancer 1980; 1(46):2074–87.

49. Baran LR, Ruben BS, Kechijian P, et al. Non-melanoma Hutchinson's sign: a reappraisal of this important, remarkable melanoma simulant. J Eur Acad Dermatol Venereol 2018;32(3):495–501.

50. Baran R, Kechijian P. Hutchinson ' s sign : a reappraisal. J Am Acad Dermatol 1996;34(1):87–90.

51. Tosti A, Baran R, Morelli R, et al. Progressive fading of longitudinal melanonychia due to a nail matrix melanocytic nevus in a child. Arch Derm 1994;130:1076–7.

52. Koga H. Dermoscopic evaluation of melanonychia. J Dermatol 2017;44(5):515–7.

53. Chiacchio ND, Farias DC, Piraccini BM, et al. Consensus on melanonychia nail plate dermoscopy. An Bras Dermatol 2013;88(2):309–13.

54. Levit EK, Kagen MH, Scher RK, et al. The ABC rule for clinical detection of subungual melanoma. J Am Acad Dermatol 2000;42:269–74.

55. Ko D, Oromendia C, Scher R, et al. Retrospective single-center study evaluating clinical and dermoscopic features of longitudinal melanonychia, ABC-DEF criteria, and risk of malignancy. J Am Acad Dermatol 2019;80(5):1272–83.

56. Lee JH, Park J, Lee JH, et al. Early detection of subungual melanoma in situ : proposal of ABCD strategy in clinical practice based on Case Series. Ann Dermatol 2018;30(1):36–40.

57. Ohn J, Jo G, Cho Y, et al. Assessment of a predictive scoring model for dermoscopy of subungual melanoma in situ. JAMA Dermatol 2018;154(8):890–6.

58. Smith RJ, Rubin AI. Pediatric nail disorders: a review. Curr Opin Pediatr 2020;32(4):506–15.

59. Mannava KA, Mannava S, Koman LA, et al. Longitudinal melanonychia: detection and management of nail melanoma. Hand Surg 2013;18(1):133–9.

60. Jellinek N. Nail matrix biopsy of longitudinal melanonychia: diagnostic algorithm including the matrix shave biopsy. J Am Acad Dermatol 2007;56(5):803–10.

61. Cordoro KM, Gupta D, Frieden IJ, et al. Pediatric melanoma: Results of a large cohort study and proposal for modified ABCD detection criteria for children. J Am Acad Dermatol 2013;68(6):913–25.

Addressing Frequently Asked Questions and Dispelling Myths About Melanocytic Nevi in Children

James Anderson-Vildósola, MD, Ángela Hernández-Martín, MD*

KEYWORDS

- Congenital melanocytic nevus • Acquired melanocytic nevus • Melanoma • Sunscreen
- Sun protection • Children

KEY POINTS

- The risk of malignancy of an isolated CMN is very low regardless of its size and location.
- The number of acquired congenital melanocytic nevus increases with age and is higher in children with lower phototypes and intense sun exposure.
- MN may clear in color and acquire volume with age, but this morphological change does not indicate malignant transformation.
- Information such as family history of melanoma or personal history of repeated sunburns can help identify which patients are at increased risk for melanoma.
- Sunscreens must be applied to the entire skin surface exposed to the sun and not only and specifically to melanocytic nevus.

INTRODUCTION

Melanocytic nevi (MN) are congenital (CMN) or acquired (AMN) benign melanocytic neoplasms. CMN are present from birth, although depending on their size and color, they may not become clinically evident until the first months of life. The incidence of CMN is estimated between 0.2% and 2.1% of newborns.[1,2] Classically, they have been divided according to the size of their diameter into small (<1.5 cm), medium (1.5–20 cm), and large (>20 cm).[3] In 2004, the giant CMN category was added to designate nevi with a diameter exceeding 40 cm.[4] CMN can present as single or multiple lesions. In the latter, there may be a larger nevus accompanied by other smaller ones (satellite CMN) or multiple lesions of similar size (multiple CMN).

AMN develop throughout time, predominantly during the first two decades of life.[5] The most common AMN are small, pigmented lesions (1–5 mm), homogeneous in color, with well-defined and regular borders. In some cases, color may be heterogeneous, but symmetry is present, and there are no additional clinical or dermoscopic concerning signs. Depending on their clinical and histologic appearance, specific subtypes are distinguished, among which are Spitz nevus and Reed nevus, typically presenting in children. Spitz nevus prevalence varies between 1.4 and 7 cases per 100,000 inhabitants, and it is characteristically a nonpigmented AMN with a reddish hue (**Fig. 1**).[6] From a histologic point of view, it is distinguished by the presence of theca of melanocytic cells of epithelioid or spindle morphology. The pigmented variant is called Reed nevus and is defined by dark-brown pigmentation and a dermoscopic starburst pattern (**Figs. 2** and **3**).[7] Another subtype of AMN is called atypical or dysplastic nevus, which, despite its benign biologic behavior, presents an alarming appearance because of its heterogeneous tone, size, and irregularity of its edges.[8] In

Department of Dermatology, Hospital Infantil Niño Jesús, Madrid, Spain
* Corresponding author. Department of Dermatology, Hospital Infantil Niño Jesús, Avda. Menéndez Pelayo 65, Madrid 28009, Spain.
E-mail address: ahernandez@aedv.es

Dermatol Clin 40 (2022) 51–59
https://doi.org/10.1016/j.det.2021.09.005

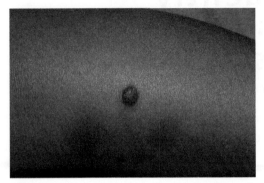

Fig. 1. Spitz nevus. Red dome-shaped papule on the lower limb of a 3-year-old boy.

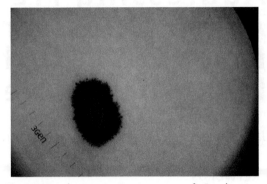

Fig. 3. Reed nevus. Dermoscopy of Reed nevus showing the classical starburst pattern.

general, dysplastic nevi are rare in childhood except in the context of dysplastic nevus syndrome, defined by the existence of a history of melanoma in one or more first- or second-degree relatives, the presence of 50 or more MN with the aforementioned "atypical" clinical appearance, and their distinctive histologic characteristics. Despite their low frequency, patients with atypical or dysplastic nevi compose a particular subgroup to consider because of their increased likelihood of developing melanoma.[9]

The reason for the appearance of MN is not precisely known. Molecular studies indicate that CMN appear as a result of somatic mutations in *NRAS* and *BRAF* genes,[10,11] whereas AMN would be mainly conditioned by mutations in *BRAF*.[12–14] Despite CMN having a similar mutational profile as melanoma,[15–17] only a tiny proportion of nevi ultimately give rise to melanoma. It is estimated that any single nevus's annual transformation rate ranges from approximately 1 in 200,000 in individuals younger than 40 years of age to approximately 1 in 33,000 if they are older than 60 years.[18]

MN appear mainly in childhood and are a cause for concern in parents and caregivers, because of the aesthetic consequences and the risk of malignant transformation, and other uncertainties based

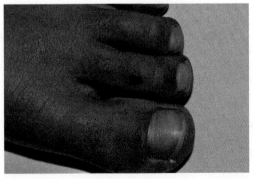

Fig. 2. Reed nevus. Hyperpigmented irregularly bordered lesion on dorsum of toe.

more on beliefs than on proper scientific evidence. In this review, we answer the most frequently asked questions posed by parents and caregivers, basing our responses on scientific evidence.

DO CONGENITAL MELANOCYTIC NEVI HAVE A HIGH RISK OF MALIGNANT TRANSFORMATION?

Although classically it has been considered that CMN had a high risk of malignant transformation, this view has largely changed over the years. In the 1970s and 1980s, it was considered that the risk of developing melanoma within a CMN was about 20%, but estimates were imprecise because of small study sizes and selection bias, which overestimated the risk.[19–21] However, subsequent series that included a more significant number of patients observed a markedly lower risk. A systematic review published in 2006 with data from 6571 patients[19] determined that the incidence varied widely depending on the sample size, ranging between 0.05% in the largest sample of 3922 cases,[1] and 10.7% in a sample of 56 cases.[20] According to this systematic review, the overall incidence of melanoma is much higher in large or giant CMN, whereas melanoma seems to be exceptional in small CMN.[19] More recently, a prospective study conducted in the United Kingdom with a cohort of 448 patients observed an overall incidence of 2.2%.[22] These authors found that the 10 patients in the study who developed melanoma had more than one CMN, whereas no patient with a single CMN, regardless of size and location, presented this outcome. However, 7 of the 10 patients who developed melanoma had a giant CMN as one of the lesions. Hence, if we exclusively consider this group of patients, melanoma incidence rises to 8%. Likewise, although there is extensive literature highlighting an elevated risk of malignant transformation of large lesions located on the central area of the back,[19,23,24] the authors found that the factor with the highest statistical power for predicting melanoma in the context of a CMN was not the size or location of the lesion, but rather the detection of a concomitant morphologic alteration in the central nervous system (CNS).[22] In turn, the latter is more likely in newborns with two or more CMN regardless of their size and location. Consequently, these authors recommend a screening MRI study of the CNS for all newborns with more than one CMN, especially if one of them is giant.[22]

The risk of malignancy of an isolated CMN is very low no matter the size or location. If the newborn has multiple CMN, and, in particular, if one of them is larger than the rest, close dermatologic and neurologic follow-up is recommended. Performing an MRI of the CNS within the first 6 months of life must be considered.

WHY DOES MY CHILD HAVE MORE AND MORE MOLES?

Patients may acquire an increasing number of MN throughout childhood, and in some patients this increase is particularly striking (**Fig. 4**). The prevalence of AMN is related to various factors including age, sex, phototype, and intensity of sunlight exposure. Concerning age, few nevi are present in early childhood, but their number increases with time, especially from 12 years of age on, reaching a peak in the third decade of life.[25,26] The difference in prevalence by sex is controversial,[27,28] but it seems the number of AMN is higher in adolescent men than in women after menarche.[29] As for skin type, individuals with a lower phototype (red hair, blue eyes, easy sunburning) tend to have a higher number of MN than individuals of darker skin phototype.[26,29]

Regarding sun exposure, it seems that the intensity of sun exposure is proportional to the number of AMN,[30,31] whether it is intermittent or continuous.[32] The beneficial effect of sunscreens during childhood in reducing the appearance of MN is controversial. A meta-analysis of the literature published in 2013 found no evidence that the use of sunscreens in childhood prevented the appearance of MN,[33] but another more recent study observed this beneficial effect if the sun protection factor (SPF) is higher than 30.[29] On the contrary, the use of sunscreens with an SPF less than 30 is related to a tendency to develop a vaster number of nevi, probably caused by the combination of insufficient protection and a false sense of security.[29]

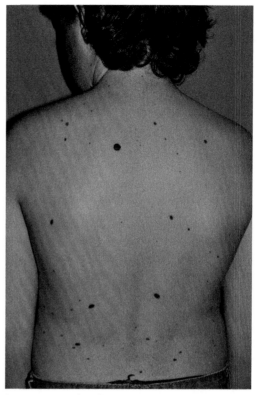

Fig. 4. Acquired melanocytic nevus. Twelve-year-old boy showing numerous acquired melanocytic nevi on the back. Note the different size, morphology, and color.

An increasing number of AMN can develop throughout childhood, especially in children with fair skin/lower phototypes and frequent or intense sun exposure.

WHAT ARE THE WARNING SIGNS THAT A MOLE IS BECOMING MALIGNANT?

The incidence of melanoma in children is much lower than in adults, and exceedingly rare in children younger than 10 years of age, so melanoma is not usually included among the main differential diagnoses in younger children. Complicating matters more, the clinical warning signs are also different, making it challenging to identify. Thus, the classic warning signs included in the acronym "ABCDE" (asymmetry, border irregularity, color variation, diameter ≥6 mm, evolution) may be absent in up to 60% of preadolescents and 40% of adolescents. In addition, because 76% of melanoma in children are amelanotic (nonpigmented) and develop as red or pink lesions, "modified ABCD" criteria have been proposed: A for amelanotic (red or pink lesion, and therefore not necessarily dark); B for "bleeding, bump" (ulceration and bulging are indicative clinical data); C for color uniformity (and not heterogeneous, as classically occurs in adult melanoma); and D for "de novo, any diameter" (without preceding lesion, of any size) (**Table 1**).[34] Another additional criterion for melanoma suspicion is the acronym EFR (elevated, firm, and growing), regarding the appearance of an elevated, firm, and growing lesion persisting for more than 1 month. The EFR rule helps exclude inflammatory lesions, such as insect bites or folliculitis, common in the pediatric population, that are usually stable and tend to resolve in less than 1 month. Unlike in adult melanoma, the lesion diameter (D of the ABCDE rule) is not a valid discrimination factor for pediatric melanoma, so the D of the modified ABCD rule for children includes lesions of any diameter.[34] Some series observed that about 50% of pediatric deaths caused by melanoma had lesions of 5 mm or less in diameter,[34–36] so the size of lesions in children does not serve to discriminate between benign and malignant neoplasms. Finally, interpreting evolution, or the E of the classic rule, is challenging in children because morphologic changes of MN throughout childhood are frequent and lack prognostic significance (**Fig. 5**).

Despite the extremely low incidence of melanoma in children, it must be kept in mind that specific subgroups of pediatric patients are at a higher risk, such as fair-skinned, blue-eyed, red-haired individuals; children with poor tanning ability and prone to sunburn; or those with a genetic predisposition (familial melanoma, xeroderma pigmentosum, or immunodeficiencies).[37]

> The classical "ABCDE" criteria are not sensitive enough in children and must be accompanied by additional clinical data adapted to the pediatric age (modified ABCD criteria). Melanomas in children younger than 10 years of age usually manifest as elevated, firm, and growing red bumps, whereas clinical signs of malignant transformation in adolescents are more likely to adapt to classical ABCDE rules. Simple information, such as a family history of melanoma or personal history of repeated sunburns, can help identify which patients are at increased risk for melanoma.

IS IT NECESSARY THAT A DERMATOLOGIST REVIEW ALL MELANOCYTIC NEVI IN CHILDREN (CONGENITAL AND ACQUIRED)?

Although it is difficult to calculate because of the high prevalence of MN in a healthy population, the estimated risk of MN becoming malignant is low, ranging from 0.0005% (or <1 in 200,000)

Table 1
Conventional ABCDE melanoma detection criteria and additional ABCD criteria for children

Conventional Criteria	Additional Criteria for Children
A Asymmetry	**A**melanotic
B Border irregularity	**B**leeding, **B**ump
C Color variation	Color uniformity
D Diameter ≥6 mm	De novo, any **D**iameter
E Evolution	EFG[a] rule

[a] Elevated, firm, and growing.

before the age of 40 years, to 0.003% (1 in 33,000).[18] In addition, melanoma arises as a de novo lesion in 70% of cases,[38,39] so it does not seem necessary to refer all patients with benign-looking MN to specialized care.

Despite this, and although the risk of melanoma within MN in the general pediatric population is low, we should not exclude beforehand such diagnostic possibility. Therefore, the previously mentioned groups at high risk of developing melanoma (ie, family history of melanoma, repeated sunburns, or immunodeficiency), any clinically suspicious lesion (according to ABCDE rules in different ages), or even one with an apparently benign morphology but that raises personal concerns about its biologic behavior, should be referred to a dermatologist.

Likewise, MN with potential relevant aesthetic impact may need a referral for a multidisciplinary approach. In particular, the deterioration in patients' quality of life because of facial skin lesions has been well studied.[40,41] Keep in mind that a significant portion of CMN undergo marked lightning throughout childhood,[42] and a "wait and see" approach may be reasonable. Nor should it be forgotten that surgical interventions, especially when the benefit is not entirely clear, can entail considerable emotional stress for the patient and parents and caregivers, and pose a risk associated with repeated surgical interventions under general anesthesia.[43,44] However, it is essential to assess each case individually, paying attention to the patients' and their parents' and caregivers' expectations, because hopes frequently do not correspond with reality, and the scar may not be as satisfactory as expected or may even be unaesthetic.[45] Along with other authors,[46] we recommend addressing surgically those facial nevi in which a potential disfiguring surgical sequelae is less than the original lesion.

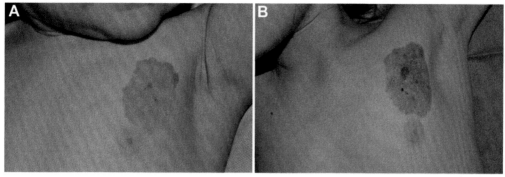

Fig. 5. Congenital melanocytic nevus. Changing appearance with time of a congenital melanocytic nevus of small-to-medium size on the trunk when the patient was 9 months old (*A*) and 10 years old (*B*).

> Children with benign-looking MN do not require routine referral to the dermatologist unless the patient is at risk of developing melanoma for any reason; has atypical-appearing, rapidly evolving, or symptomatic nevi; or has a nevus requiring a multidisciplinary approach because of its aesthetic impact.

ARE MELANOCYTIC NEVI ON THE PALMS AND SOLES MORE DANGEROUS THAN THOSE IN OTHER LOCATIONS?

There is a widely held belief that MN in palms and soles have a higher risk of malignant transformation than those in other parts of the body, but current evidence does not support this. Acral melanomas are the least common type in the United States, representing 2% to 3% of all melanomas.[47] Acral melanomas are the most prevalent group in Japan, where they account for 47% of all melanomas.[48] Although in the White population the risk of suffering a melanoma is directly proportional to the total number of AMN, the number of AMN present in Japanese individuals' soles does not seem to be a risk factor for suffering acral melanoma.[49] Hence, in a study of 104 Japanese patients with acral melanoma, not only did less than 11% of patients have a previous MN at that location, but the number of acral MN was not higher in people with acral melanoma than the rest of the population.[50] Another study compared the topographic distribution of acral MN with melanomas at this location, finding a different distribution of the locations of MN and acral melanomas.[48] Acral melanomas in the Japanese population appear de novo, without preceding MN, in almost 90% of cases and arise in a different location from where acral MN usually appear.[48] In addition, the mutational profile of palmar and plantar MN is similar to MN located elsewhere on the body,[48,50] whereas the mutations

of acral melanomas are different from those of acral nevi, ruling out a potential association.[51,52]

> There is no current evidence to support the belief that acral MN have a more aggressive biologic behavior than MN in other locations, so their diagnosis, management, and monitoring should be similar to that of lesions in other locations.

HOW OFTEN SHOULD MELANOCYTIC NEVI BE CHECKED?

Patients with increased risk of melanoma should be reviewed periodically, along with clinical and dermoscopic follow-up of doubtful lesions, but it is uncertain what approach to take for children with CMN and AMN in the absence of warning signs. Many experts recommend an annual check-up of MN, whereas others suggest that patients request a follow-up visit only if they observe morphologic changes or discomfort in any of the lesions. Nevertheless, there is no scientific evidence to support the former, nor does self-examination seem reliable enough.[53] Traditionally, the classic ABCDE rule has been emphasized to teach how to detect worrisome MN,[54] but these warning signs may have limited utility in the pediatric age.[34] In our practice, we do not routinely review CMN or AMN when their clinical and dermoscopic characteristics are banal, but we recommend a follow-up visit in the event of any morphologic change or new-onset symptoms.

> There is no well-defined universal strategy with sufficient evidence to make recommendations on the specific need to review MN with benign characteristics in children with no risk factors for melanoma or on the ideal timing of such reviews.

IS IT BETTER TO BE "SAFE THAN SORRY"? (IS IT ADVISABLE TO REMOVE AS MANY NEVI AS POSSIBLE AS SOON AS POSSIBLE?)

There is strong evidence that the number of AMN is a significant risk factor for the development of melanoma,[27,28] but the effectiveness of surgical excision as a preventive measure is more than doubtful. It is logical to think that the greater the number of melanocytes, the greater the risk of malignant transformation of these cells, and therefore, the prophylactic surgical removal of MN would, in theory, have a potential therapeutic value. However, the question is whether this attitude is cost-effective, something that has not been proved useful in young individuals so far.[55]

The risk of malignancy in solitary CMN is low, regardless of their size and location. Moreover, a substantial number of patients develop melanoma outside of CMN,[19] so theoretically, complete removal of the lesion would not eliminate the risk. Besides, there are cases where melanoma appeared where a CMN had previously been partially or entirely removed.[56] Consequently, the excision of CMN does not eliminate the risk of melanoma.[19] Regarding the theoretic possibility of malignancy of AMN, calculating the percentage of malignancy is complex because of the latter's high prevalence; however, only 30% of melanomas appear on previous AMN.[38,39] Accordingly, most of them would be de novo lesions, and prophylactic removal of AMN would not be beneficial.

> There is no scientific evidence to support prophylactic removal of either AMN or CMN, and therefore, surgery would only be advocated if there are clinical findings to advise it.

ARE NEVI THAT BULGE WORRISOME?

Often, patients come to our office expressing their desire to remove exophytic lesions on the body, mostly on their trunk or scalp. The motivations are diverse, but in general, aesthetic criteria prevail and, secondarily, the discomfort caused by rubbing against clothing or during hairstyling. Descriptions of the natural progression of AMN pointing to their natural evolution toward elevation date back to the nineteenth century.[57] This slow elevation from a nearly flat to raised lesion occurs because of the migration of melanocytes to deeper regions of the dermis, "lifting" the overlying tissue and producing a color lightning, which can become pink without evidence of pigmentation (**Fig. 6**).[57–59] Importantly, in most cases, this slow progression is not worrisome. Unless the lesion is symptomatic or subject to repeated trauma by brushes or clothing, otherwise banal-appearing lesions that are raised do not require removal.

> MN are changing lesions in changing individuals, and not all morphologic changes reflect malignant transformation. MN may clear in color and acquire volume with age, but this morphologic change does not indicate malignant transformation.

HOW CAN I PREVENT MALIGNANT TRANSFORMATION OF MOLES?

Intense sun exposure is a well-known risk factor for developing skin cancer. In particular, melanoma development is strongly related to repeated sunburns during childhood and adolescence, and therefore, implementing the appropriate strategies for sun protection is essential. However, a study performed in 2013 demonstrated that only 10% of students between 14 and 17 years of age applied sunscreen with an SPF greater than or equal to 15 while performing outdoor activities.[60] Younger children are prone to use sunscreens properly because their parents and caregivers take on the responsibility to apply them regularly. However, the adherence to sun protection diminishes noticeably with age. For example, a study performed in the United States observed that 69% of adolescents aged between 11 and 18 years had experienced sunburn the previous summer.[61]

Physicians and school policies play a crucial role in educational interventions to promote sun-protective behaviors, but, most interestingly, only 44% of adolescents and their parents reported receiving advice on photoprotection from their physicians, whereas only 22% of physicians acknowledged giving recommendations on the subject to their patients.[62] A recent survey among pediatricians showed that sun protection ranked low among preventive topics

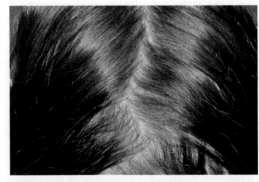

Fig. 6. Raised acquired pink melanocytic nevus on the scalp in a 14-year-old girl. The lesion was excised because of repeated traumatization of the lesion during hair styling.

and that only a minority of them offered to counsel about sun protection and indoor tanning.[63]

These data show that educational interventions in sun protection behaviors have ample room for improvement.[64]

Although the risk of malignant transformation of an individual MN is low, appropriate sun protection from an early age is important in minimizing this risk. Caregivers and parents play a pivotal role, and improvement of educational interventions carried out by physicians and health care providers is needed.

WHICH IS THE BEST SUNSCREEN?

The importance of proper use of topical sunscreens in childhood to prevent the cumulative effect of solar radiation (UVA and UVB) on the skin is well known to parents and caregivers and raises a recurring question about the ideal product. Sunscreens contain chemical (organic) or physical (inorganic) compounds that block ultraviolet radiation. In general, physical or inorganic sunscreens are preferred in children to minimize the risks of sensitization and toxicity.[65] The SPF, broad-spectrum activity against UVA and UVB, the amount of sunscreen applied, and the regularity of application are essential factors determining the usefulness of a sunscreen's protective effects.

The SPF only measures UVB protection (not UVA) and is not a measure of time but a measure of the fraction of sunburn-producing UV rays that reach the skin. For example, "SPF 20" means that one-twentieth of the burning radiation will reach the skin.[66] The American Academy of Dermatology recommends using SPF sunscreens equal to or greater than 30 regardless of skin type.[67] It is important to use sunscreen with broad-spectrum activity. The amount of protective cream is another element that determines its effectiveness, which is proportional to the amount applied. A study carried out with primary school children aged 5 to 12 years who applied the sunscreen themselves found that they used less than half of the recommended 2 g/cm^2.[68] Finally, regular reapplication of the sun protection cream, especially after bathing and physical exercise, optimizes its sustained effect throughout the photo-exposure period. The American Academy of Dermatology recommends reapplying sunscreen approximately every 2 hours, or after swimming or sweating, according to the directions on the bottle.[67] Sun protection strategies in addition to the correct use of sunscreens include photoprotective clothing and sunglasses, and avoiding intense sunlight at peak hours of UV radiation.

The best sunscreen is the one that you apply in enough quantity and frequency (again and again). Ensure your sunscreen offers broad-spectrum protection (blocks UVA and UVB radiation) and has a minimum SPF of 30.

CLINICS CARE POINTS

- The risk of malignancy of a solitary congenital melanocytic nevus is low, regardless of its size and location.
- The number of acquired melanocytic nevi increases throughout childhood, especially in children with lower phototypes and those who are more exposed to the sun, particularly if repeated sunburns.
- Surgical management of melanocytic nevi does not prevent melanoma and must be discussed individually.
- Melanoma is extremely rare in children younger than 10 years of age and may be challenging to recognize. The classic "ABCDE" alarm criteria for early detection of melanoma are not sensitive enough in children and must be accompanied by additional clinical information and pediatric-related criteria.
- Sunscreens must be applied to the entire skin surface exposed to the sun and not only and specifically to melanocytic nevi. Clothing, hats, and sunglasses offer additional protection.
- Physicians and school policies play a key role in educational interventions to promote sun-protective behaviors to prevent skin cancer.

DISCLOSURE

Dr J. Anderson-Vildósola has no conflict of interest to declare. Dr A. Hernández-Martín has conducted clinical trials for Mayne Pharma and Celgene; and has received honoraria for academic lectures from Viatrix, Leti Pharma, Pierre Fabre, and Beiersdorf Laboratories.

REFERENCES

1. Berg P, Lindelöf B. Congenital melanocytic naevi and cutaneous melanoma. Melanoma Res 2003;13:441–5.
2. Rivers JK, Frederiksen PC, Dibdin C. A prevalence survey of dermatoses in the Australian neonate. J Am Acad Dermatol 1990;23:77–81.
3. Kopf AW, Bart RS, Hennessey P. Congenital nevocytic nevi and malignant melanomas. J Am Acad Dermatol 1979;1:123–30.

4. Krengel S, Scope A, Dusza SW, et al. New recommendations for the categorization of cutaneous features of congenital melanocytic nevi. J Am Acad Dermatol 2013;68:441–51.

5. Crane LA, Mokrohisky ST, Dellavalle RP, et al. Melanocytic nevus development in Colorado children born in 1998: a longitudinal study. Arch Dermatol 2009;145:148–56.

6. Dika E, Ravaioli GM, Fanti PA, et al. Spitz nevi and other spitzoid neoplasms in children: overview of incidence data and diagnostic criteria. Pediatr Dermatol 2017;34:25–32.

7. Requena L, Yus ES. Pigmented spindle cell naevus. Br J Dermatol 1990;123:757–63.

8. Rosendahl CO, Grant-Kels JM, Que SKT. Dysplastic nevus: fact and fiction. J Am Acad Dermatol 2015;73:507–12.

9. Goldsmith LA, Askin FB, Chang AE, et al. Diagnosis and treatment of early melanoma: NIH consensus development panel on early melanoma. JAMA 1992;268:1314–9.

10. Charbel C, Fontaine RH, Malouf GG, et al. NRAS mutation is the sole recurrent somatic mutation in large congenital melanocytic nevi. J Invest Dermatol 2014;134:1067–74.

11. Kinsler VA, Thomas AC, Ishida M, et al. Multiple congenital melanocytic nevi and neurocutaneous melanosis are caused by postzygotic mutations in codon 61 of NRAS. J Invest Dermatol 2013;133:2229–36.

12. Poynter JN, Elder JT, Fullen DR, et al. BRAF and NRAS mutations in melanoma and melanocytic nevi. Melanoma Res 2006;16:267–73.

13. Wu J, Rosenbaum E, Begum S, et al. Distribution of BRAF T1799A(V600E) mutations across various types of benign nevi: implications for melanocytic tumorigenesis. Am J Dermatopathol 2007;29:534–7.

14. Ichii-Nakato N, Takata M, Takayanagi S, et al. High frequency of BRAFV600E mutation in acquired nevi and small congenital nevi, but low frequency of mutation in medium-sized congenital nevi. J Invest Dermatol 2006;126:2111–8.

15. Ball NJ, Yohn JJ, Morelli JG, et al. RAS mutations in human melanoma: a marker of malignant progression. J Invest Dermatol 1994;102:285–90.

16. van 't Veer LJ, Burgering BM, Versteeg R, et al. N-ras mutations in human cutaneous melanoma from sun-exposed body sites. Mol Cell Biol 1989;9:3114–6.

17. Davies H, Bignell GR, Cox C, et al. Mutations of the BRAF gene in human cancer. Nature 2002;417:949–54.

18. Tsao H, Bevona C, Goggins W, et al. The transformation rate of moles (melanocytic nevi) into cutaneous melanoma: a population-based estimate. Arch Dermatol 2003;139:282–8.

19. Krengel S, Hauschild A, Schafer T. Melanoma risk in congenital melanocytic naevi: a systematic review. Br J Dermatol 2006;155:1–8.

20. Greely PW, Middleton AG, Curtin JW. Incidence of malignancy in giant pigmented nevi. Plast Recontr Surg 1977;36:26–37.

21. Quaba AA, Wallace AF. The incidence of malignant melanoma (0 to 15 years of age) arising in 'large' congenital nevocellular nevi. Plast Recontr Surg 1986;78:174–81.

22. Kinsler VA, O'Hare P, Bulstrode N, et al. Melanoma in congenital melanocytic naevi. Br J Dermatol 2017; 176:1131–43.

23. Kinsler VA, Chong WK, Aylett SE, et al. Complications of congenital melanocytic naevi in children: analysis of 16 years' experience and clinical practice. Br J Dermatol 2008;159:907–14.

24. Ka VSK, Dusza SW, Halpern AC, et al. The association between large congenital melanocytic naevi and cutaneous melanoma: preliminary findings from an Internet-based registry of 379 patients. Melanoma Res 2005;15:61–7.

25. Siskind V, Darlington S, Green L, et al. Evolution of melanocytic nevi on the faces and necks of adolescents: a 4 y longitudinal study. J Invest Dermatol 2002;118:500–4.

26. Luther H, Altmeyer P, Garbe C, et al. Increase of melanocytic nevus counts in children during 5 years of follow-up and analysis of associated factors. Arch Dermatol 1996;132:1473–8.

27. Bataille V, Bishop J, Sasieni P, et al. Risk of cutaneous melanoma in relation to the numbers, types and sites of naevi: a case-control study. Br J Cancer 1996;73:1605–11.

28. Grulich AE, Bataille V, Swerdlow AJ, et al. Naevi and pigmentary characteristics as risk factors for melanoma in a high-risk population: a case-control study in New South Wales, Australia. Int J Cancer 1996;67(4):485-91.

29. De Giorgi V, Gori A, Greco A, et al. Sun-protection behavior, pubertal development and menarche: factors influencing the melanocytic nevi development: the results of an observational study of 1,512 children. J Invest Dermatol 2018;138:2144–51.

30. Baron AE, Asdigian NL, Gonzalez V, et al. Interactions between ultraviolet light and MC1R and OCA2 variants are determinants of childhood nevus and freckle phenotypes. Cancer Epidemiol Biomarkers Prev 2014;23:2829–39.

31. Dulon M, Weichenthal M, Blettner M, et al. Sun exposure and number of nevi in 5- to 6-year-old European children. J Clin Epidemiol 2002;55:1075–81.

32. Asdigian NL, Barón AE, Morelli JG, et al. Trajectories of nevus development from age 3 to 16 years in the colorado kids sun care program cohort. JAMA Dermatol 2018;154:1272.

33. de Maleissye M-F, Beauchet A, Saiag P, et al. Sunscreen use and melanocytic nevi in children: a systematic review: sunscreen and nevi in children. Pediatr Dermatol 2013;30:51–9.

34. Cordoro KM, Gupta D, Frieden IJ, et al. Pediatric melanoma: results of a large cohort study and proposal for modified ABCD detection criteria for children. J Am Acad Dermatol 2013;68:913–25.

35. Downard CD, Rapkin LB, Gow KW. Melanoma in children and adolescents. Surg Oncol 2007;16(3):215-20.

36. Melnik M, Urdaneta L, Al-Jurf A, et al. Malignant melanoma in childhood and adolescence. Am Surg 1986;52:142–7.
37. Childhood melanoma treatment (PDQ®): health professional version. In: PDQ cancer information summaries. Bethesda, MD: National Cancer Institute (US); 2002.
38. Lin WM, Luo S, Muzikansky A, et al. Outcome of patients with de novo versus nevus-associated melanoma. J Am Acad Dermatol 2015;72:54–8.
39. Bevona C. Cutaneous melanomas associated with nevi. Arch Dermatol 2003;139:1620.
40. Masnari O, Neuhaus K, Aegerter T, et al. Predictors of Health-related Quality of Life and Psychological Adjustment in Children and Adolescents With Congenital Melanocytic Nevi: Analysis of Parent Reports. J Pediatr Psychol. 2019;44(6):714-725.
41. Brown MM, Chamlin SL, Smidt AC. Quality of life in pediatric dermatology. Dermatol Clin 2013;31:211–21.
42. Margileth AM. Spontaneous regression of large congenital melanocytic nevi, with a halo rim in 17 children with large scalp and trunk nevi during 45 years: a review of the literature. Clin Pediatr (Phila) 2019;58:313–9.
43. Loepke AW, Soriano SG. An assessment of the effects of general anesthetics on developing brain structure and neurocognitive function. Anesth Analg 2008;106:1681–707.
44. Ben-Ari A, Margalit D, Nachshoni L, et al. Traumatic stress among children after surgical intervention for congenital melanocytic nevi: a pilot study. Dermatol Surg 2019. https://doi.org/10.1097/DSS.0000000000002276.
45. Ruiz-Maldonado R, Tamayo L, Laterza AM, et al. Giant pigmented nevi: clinical, histopathologic, and therapeutic considerations. J Pediatr 1992;120:906–11.
46. Kinsler V, Bulstrode N. The role of surgery in the management of congenital melanocytic naevi in children: a perspective from Great Ormond Street Hospital. J Plast Reconstr Aesthet Surg 2009;62(5):595-601.
47. Bradford PT, Goldstein AM, McMaster ML, et al. Acral lentiginous melanoma: incidence and survival patterns in the United States, 1986-2005. Arch Dermatol 2009;145:8.
48. Ghanavatian S, Costello CM, Buras MR, et al. Density and distribution of acral melanocytic nevi and acral melanomas on the plantar surface of the foot. J Am Acad Dermatol 2019;80:790–2.e2.
49. Rokuhara S, Saida T, Oguchi M, et al. Number of acquired melanocytic nevi in patients with melanoma and control subjects in Japan: nevus count is a significant risk factor for nonacral melanoma but not for acral melanoma. J Am Acad Dermatol 2004;50:695–700.
50. Kogushi-Nishi H, Kawasaki J, Kageshita T, et al. The prevalence of melanocytic nevi on the soles in the Japanese population. J Am Acad Dermatol 2009;60:767–71.
51. Curtin JA, Patel HN, Cho K-H, et al. Distinct sets of genetic alterations in melanoma. N Engl J Med 2005;353(20):2135–47.
52. Sakaizawa K, Ashida A, Uchiyama A, et al. Clinical characteristics associated with BRAF, NRAS and KIT mutations in Japanese melanoma patients. J Dermatol Sci 2015;80:33–7.
53. US Preventive Services Task Force, Bibbins-Domingo K, Grossman DC, et al. Screening for skin cancer: US preventive services task force recommendation statement. JAMA 2016;316:429.
54. Weinstock M, Risica P, Martin R, et al. Melanoma early detection with thorough skin self-examination: the "check it out" randomized trial. Am J Prev Med 2007;32:517–24.
55. Waldmann A, Nolte S, Geller AC, et al. Frequency of excisions and yields of malignant skin tumors in a population-based screening intervention of 360,288 whole-body examinations. Arch Dermatol 2012;148:903–10.
56. Bett BJ. Large or multiple congenital melanocytic nevi: occurrence of neurocutaneous melanocytosis in 1008 persons. J Am Acad Dermatol 2006;54:767–77.
57. Stegmaier OC. Natural regression of the melanocytic nevus. J Invest Dermatol 1959;32:413–21.
58. Unna PG. The histopathology of the diseases of the skin. Translated from the German, with the assistance of the author, by Norman Walker. New York: Macmillan Publishing Co; 1896.
59. Stegmaier OC, Montgomery H. Histopathologic studies of pigmented nevi in children. J Invest Dermatol 1953;20:51–64.
60. Dietrich AJ. Sun protection counseling for children: primary care practice patterns and effect of an intervention on clinicians. Arch Fam Med 2000;9:155–9.
61. Cokkinides V, Weinstock M, Glanz K, et al. Trends in sunburns, sun protection practices, and attitudes toward sun exposure protection and tanning among US adolescents, 1998-2004. Pediatrics 2006;118:853–64.
62. Balk SJ. Counseling parents and children on sun protection: a national survey of pediatricians. Pediatrics 2004;114:1056–64.
63. Balk SJ, Gottschlich EA, Holman DM, et al. Counseling on sun protection and indoor tanning. Pediatrics 2017;140:e20171680.
64. Guy GPJ, Holman DM, Watson M. The important role of schools in the prevention of skin cancer. JAMA Dermatol 2016;152:1083–4.
65. Paller AS, Hawk JLM, Honig P, et al. New insights about infant and toddler skin: implications for sun protection. Pediatrics 2011;128:92–102.
66. Cripps DJ, Hegedus S. Protection factor of sunscreens to monochromatic radiation. Arch Dermatol 1974;109:202–4.
67. American Academy of Dermatology Association. SUNSCREEN FAQS [WWW document]. Available at: www.aad.org/media/stats-sunscreen. Accessed January 10, 2021.
68. Diaz A, Neale RE, Kimlin MG, et al. The children and sunscreen study: a crossover trial investigating children's sunscreen application thickness and the influence of age and dispenser type. Arch Dermatol 2012;148:606–12.

Epidermal Nevi: What Is New

Andrea R. Waldman, MD[a], Maria C. Garzon, MD[b], Kimberly D. Morel, MD[b],*

KEYWORDS

- Epidermal nevus • Epidermal nevus syndrome • Nevus sebaceous • Nevus sebaceous syndrome
- RASopathy

KEY POINTS

- When epidermal nevus syndromes are suspected, genetic evaluation plays an important role because the specific mutation may harbor clues to the associated extracutaneous manifestations.
- The clinical manifestations of epidermal nevi directly result from somatic postzygotic genetic mutations in utero, and many novel mutations have been elucidated in recent years.
- Targeted therapies are emerging as more becomes known about the genetics of EN and ENS.

INTRODUCTION

Epidermal nevi are a group of hamartomatous lesions, often congenital, characterized by hyperplasia of epidermal cells. The cells residing in the epidermis include keratinocytes, smooth muscle and adnexal cells (sebaceous, eccrine, and apocrine glands), and those comprising the hair follicles. Division into 2 categories based on their primary cell type as keratinocytic nevi and adnexal nevi has characterized these lesions.[1,2] Like other types of "birthmarks," epidermal nevi represent somatic mosaicism within the skin. With the availability of next-generation sequencing and easy accessibility of these tissues, there has been an increased understanding of the pathogenesis of epidermal nevi, which has improved classification and elucidated potential targeted therapies.[3] Moreover, we have gained an improved understanding of the relationship between specific epidermal nevi and their associated extracutaneous manifestations. This article details the clinical findings of epidermal nevi and their associated genetic syndromes and provides an update on the genetic characteristics of this heterogeneous group of skin lesions (**Fig. 1**, **Table 1**).

PATHOGENESIS

The clinical manifestations of epidermal nevi result from genetic mutations or epigenetic transformation impacting cell expression during postzygotic embryologic development in utero; this results in mosaicism in the individual, which is characterized by the presence of 2 or more genetically different cell populations by the time of birth.[4] The relationship between genotype and phenotype is complex because many distinct genetic abnormalities may lead to a similar phenotype. Furthermore, one genetic abnormality can lead to many different phenotypic presentations. Earlier timing of the postzygotic mutation tends to portend more extensive cutaneous and/or extracutaneous involvement.[4]

EPIDERMAL NEVI (KERATINOCYTIC NEVI)

Epidermal nevi, characterized by epidermal hyperplasia, often present at birth or within the first few years of life. Typically, these lesions initially present as a linear tan patch or plaque along Blaschko lines. Epidermal nevi often evolve to become darker, thicker, and more verrucous during puberty, and thus patients often present for

[a] Department of Dermatology and Pediatrics, Mount Sinai Icahn School of Medicine, 5 East 98th Street, New York, NY 10029, USA; [b] Departments of Dermatology and Pediatrics, Vagelos College of Physicians & Surgeons, Columbia University Medical Center, 161 Fort Washington Avenue, 12th Floor, New York, NY 10032, USA
* Corresponding author. 161 Fort Washington Avenue, 12th Floor, New York, NY 10032.
E-mail address: km208@cumc.columbia.edu

Dermatol Clin 40 (2022) 61–71
https://doi.org/10.1016/j.det.2021.09.006
0733-8635/22/© 2021 Elsevier Inc. All rights reserved.

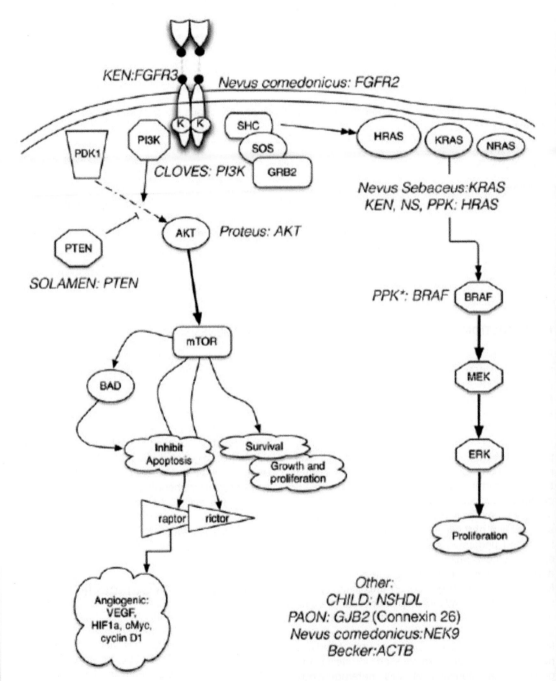

Fig. 1. Affected pathways with associated syndromes. (*Reprint with permission from Asch S, Sugarman JL. Epidermal nevus syndromes: New insights into whorls and swirls. Pediatr Dermatol. 2018 Jan;35(1):21-29.*)

evaluation during this time period. A single lesion is most common; however, large or multiple lesions may occur and herald extracutaneous involvement.

Histologically, the most common forms of keratinocytic epidermal nevi are characterized by hyperkeratosis and papillomatosis similar to seborrheic keratosis, therefore clinicopathologic correlation is required. The development of malignant tumors within keratinocytic epidermal nevi is extremely rare.[5–7] Several mutations have been demonstrated in epidermal nevi, including FGFR3, PIK3CA, HRAS, KRAS, and NRAS.[8–10]

PIK3CA, specifically the E545 G codon mosaic mutation, has been associated with epidermal nevi. This exact mutation has also been linked to

Table 1
Epidermal nevi and their associated genetic syndromes

Lesion	Pathogenic Genetic Variant
Keratinocytic nevi	
Epidermal nevus	FGFR3
	FGFR2
	HRAS
	KRAS
	NRAS
	PIK3CA
Epidermolytic ichthyosis	KRT1
	KRT10
	KRT2
CHILD syndrome	NSDHL
PTEN nevus	PTEN
Proteus syndrome and epidermal nevi	AKT1
PIK3CA-related overgrowth spectrum/CLOVES	PIK3CA
Acantholytic dyskeratotic epidermal nevus	ATP2A2
	GJB2
Inflammatory linear verrucous epidermal nevus	Not identified to date
Adnexal nevi	
Nevus sebaceous/nevus sebaceous syndrome	FGFR2
	HRAS
	KRAS
	NRAS
Porokeratotic adnexal ostial nevus	GJB2 (connexin 26)
Nevus comedonicus/nevus comedonicus syndrome	NEK9
	FGFR2
Becker nevus/Becker nevus syndrome	ACTB (beta-actin)

Abbreviations: CHILD, congenital hemidysplasia with ichthyosiform erythroderma and limb defects; CLOVES, congenital lipomatous overgrowth and vascular and skeletal anomalies

seborrheic keratoses and colorectal cancer, which highlights the importance of other factors that govern ultimate phenotype.[8] Similarly, approximately one-third of epidermal nevi have a somatic heterozygous postzygotic activating mutation in the FGFR3 oncogene, which has also been documented in association with seborrheic keratosis.[9,11]

Treatment of epidermal nevi depends on the clinical context. Epidermal nevi without functional, symptomatic, or social implications may be observed clinically. In cases in which treatment is desired or necessary, full thickness excision is definitive but may not be possible for all lesions. Other superficial destructive and topical therapies such as cryotherapy, dermabrasion, and electrodessication have been performed but recurrence is extremely common. CO_2 ablative laser therapy has been used with variable results, but recurrence, hypopigmentation, and scarring may occur.[12,13]

What Is New

- RAS oncogene mutations (HRAS most common) and FGFR2 mutations have been noted in epidermal nevi.[14,15]
- Topical sirolimus, which targets the mTOR pathway, was found to reduce the thickness of the skin lesions in a pediatric patient with a mosaic mutation in FGFR3.[16]

UNIQUE VARIANTS OF KERATINOCYTIC EPIDERMAL NEVI
Epidermolytic Ichthyosis

One unique pattern displayed by some epidermal nevi is characterized by clumping of keratin filaments in the suprabasilar cells, known as epidermolytic hyperkeratosis (EHK) and suggests a mosaic disorder of keratin 1 and 10 genes. This EHK pattern has also been reported in nevus comedonicus and porokeratotic adnexal ostial nevus (POAN) (see later sections). This pattern heralds the potential to pass on widespread epidermolytic ichthyosis, an autosomal dominant disorder, to future offspring through germline mutations. For the purpose of genetic counseling and risk stratifying, a biopsy of epidermal nevus tissue is often considered, with careful attention to the histologic features for EHK pattern.[17]

What is new and what is noteworthy

- Epidermolytic epidermal nevi resulting from somatic heterozygous mutation in KRT2 have been reported, expanding the genotypic spectrum of this subset of epidermal nevi.[18]
- Genetic counseling is recommended when the EHK pattern is seen in a nevus.[17]

Inflammatory Linear Verrucous Epidermal Nevi

Inflammatory linear verrucous epidermal nevi (ILVEN) represent a distinct variant of epidermal nevi presenting as a linear inflammatory plaque with erythema, verrucous changes, and scaling. These plaques appear most commonly on the extremities within the first 4 years of life and have a characteristic chronic course with intermittent intense inflammation. The genetic cause of ILVEN has been elusive to date, and there are no known extracutaneous associations. ILVEN are highly resistant to treatment and topical therapy with corticosteroids, and other therapies have only temporarily reduced inflammation.[19] Treatment success with systemic and/or biologic therapy has been documented when co-occurring with psoriasis. Among these therapies are etanercept, adalimumab, and thalidomide.[20–22] Excision and skin grafts may be considered for select lesions.[23] Improvement in inflammation has been reported with topical sirolimus.[24] Topical crisaborole has also been reported to resolve pruritus and improve erythema and thickness in a pediatric patient with ILVEN.[25]

Acantholytic Dyskeratotic Epidermal Nevus

Acantholytic dyskeratotic epidermal nevus (ADEN) is a rare and distinct subtype of epidermal nevi characterized by its unique histologic pattern of "Darier-like" acantholysis and dyskeratosis.[26] Several reports of postzygotic somatic ATP2A2 mutations localized to ADEN tissue have been reported. ATP2A2, also implicated as the defective gene in Darier disease, encodes the sarcoplasmic/endoplasmic reticulum Ca(2+) ATPase isoform 2 (SERCA2).[27,28] A novel somatic mutation

in GJB2 gene, encoding connexin 26, has also been reported in ADEN.[29]

What is new

- Genetic testing for ATP2A2 and GJB2 and/or immunohistochemical staining for SERCA2 protein expression within epidermal nevi tissue may be considered with clinicopathologic correlation.[29,30]

Syndromes Associated with Keratinocytic Epidermal Nevi

Epidermal nevus syndromes are characterized by the presence of epidermal nevi in addition to extracutaneous organ involvement including neurologic, ophthalmologic, and skeletal findings. The presence of certain types and clinical characteristics of epidermal nevi may therefore warrant further investigation. Several syndromes have been described and are discussed in the following section.

CONGENITAL HEMIDYSPLASIA WITH ICHTHYOSIFORM ERYTHRODERMA AND LIMB DEFECTS) SYNDROME

Congenital hemidysplasia with ichthyosiform erythroderma and limb defects (CHILD) syndrome is a rare condition with variable clinical expression characterized by an epidermal nevus or nevi in association with multiple ipsilateral extracutaneous features including skeletal, neurologic, cardiac, pulmonary, and renal anomalies in affected females. This condition arises in females only as a result of an X-linked dominant loss-of-function mutation, which is lethal in males. The mutation occurs in the NSDHL gene, encoding 3B-hydroxysteroid dehydrogenase, which is involved in cholesterol metabolism.[31,32]

NOTEWORTHY THERAPEUTICS

- Because CHILD syndrome is a lipid metabolic disorder, a novel pathogenesis-based therapy using topically applied lovastatin or simvastatin and cholesterol lotion has been successful in treating the cutaneous lesions of patients with CHILD syndrome.[33–35]

Proteus Syndrome and Epidermal Nevi

Proteus syndrome, a progressive disorder characterized by segmental or mosaic patchy and asymmetric cutaneous and extracutaneous tissue overgrowth, results from a mosaic activating mutation of the AKT1 oncogene encoding AKT1 kinase.[36–40] The AKT1 oncogene mutation causes constitutive activation of the AKT1 kinase resulting in stimulation of the AKT/phosphatidylinositol-3-kinase (PI3K) pathway and uncontrolled cell proliferation and decreased apoptosis. This pathogenic genetic change is present in varying levels across many tissue types, resulting in a broad array of tissue overgrowth in addition to tumor predisposition.[37,40,41] Epidermal nevi, vascular malformations, dysregulation of adipose tissue (lipomas and lipohypoplasia), and patchy dermal hypoplasia are common cutaneous findings.[42] Linear epidermal nevus, present in up to 50% of patients, is often not the presenting sign of Proteus syndrome but rather a clue to the clinical diagnosis. The most specific skin finding associated with Proteus syndrome is the cerebriform connective tissue nevus, typically found on the soles or palms. These lesions evolve over time along with the phenotypic progressive overgrowth, typically between 6 and 24 months of age.[43] The most common potentially fatal association of Proteus syndrome is thromboembolism.[43,44]

What Is New

- Consider *AKT1* screening as a part of genetic tissue evaluation of epidermal nevi.[45]
- A targeted AKT inhibitor, miransertib, is under study for the treatment of Proteus.[46]

LINEAR OR TYPE 2 SEGMENTAL COWDEN DISEASE (PTEN NEVUS)

Linear Cowden disease or linear PTEN nevus were terms coined in 2007 by Happle,[47] describing epidermal nevi resulting from pathogenic changes in the PTEN gene at the germline level. Neurologic associations include macrocephaly and developmental delay. Clinicians should monitor for other disorders associated with PTEN mutations, including thyroid abnormalities, breast carcinoma, gastrointestinal hamartomas, and uterine leiomyomas.[48]

PIK3CA-RELATED OVERGROWTH SPECTRUM

PIK3CA-related overgrowth spectrum (PROS), a group of segmental overgrowth syndromes resulting from somatic activating mutations in the phosphatidylinositol-3-kinase (PIK3CA)/AKT/mTOR pathway, are characterized by heterogeneous segmental overgrowth in association with cutaneous, vascular, neurologic, and/or visceral abnormalities.[49] Congenital lipomatous overgrowth and vascular and skeletal anomalies (CLOVES) syndrome is encompassed within the umbrella of PROS and is characterized by linear epidermal nevi in addition to complex progressive vascular anomalies, adipose tissue defects,

orthopedic and central nervous system (CNS) abnormalities, and epilepsy.[50–52] Growing evidence suggests that epidermal nevi arising in patients with these syndromes represent a cutaneous manifestation of the same mutations causing the overgrowth.[49]

What Is New

- Oral sirolimus has been reported for use in patients with CLOVES.[53]
- Targeted therapy with alpelisib, an inhibitor of PI3K, is under study for PIK3CA-related overgrowth syndromes.[54]

EPIDERMAL NEVI WITH HYPOPHOSPHATEMIC RICKETS (CUTANEOUS SKELETAL HYPOPHOSPHATEMIA SYNDROME)

The occurrence of epidermal nevi in association with hypophosphatemic rickets was first reported in 1969.[55] The association has been noted in several syndromes including epidermal nevus syndrome (ENS), nevus sebaceous (NS) syndrome (NSS), PPK, and PAON (see later sections), and RAS mutations have been implicated.[56] High levels of fibroblast growth factor 23 (FGF23), a hormone originating in the bone involved in the homeostasis of phosphate, have since been noted in patients with ENS associated with hypophosphatemic rickets. This hormonal signaling in excess leads to renal phosphate wasting and chronic hypophosphatemia and may result in rickets and osteomalacia in addition to other skeletal abnormalities.[57] Calcitriol and phosphate supplements are treatment modalities,[58] and surgical excision of the epidermal nevi has been reported to ameliorate the condition.[59]

What Is New

- Burosumab, an FGF23-blocking antibody, may represent a future therapeutic direction for hypophosphatemic rickets in association with epidermal nevi.[60]

NEVUS SEBACEOUS AND NEVUS SEBACEOUS SYNDROME

Nevus sebaceous (NS), also known as nevus sebaceous of Jadassohn, is a common birthmark and the prototypical "organoid nevus" because it may include multiple skin components including epidermis, sebaceous glands, hair follicles, apocrine glands, and connective tissue.[61] NS is usually noted at birth as a yellow-orange to pink, smooth or cobblestoned, linear or oval alopecic plaque most often on the scalp, but it may also arise on the face and neck. During puberty, NS tends to become more raised and verrucous, thought to be secondary to androgen stimulation of sebaceous glands.[62] Most cases of NS are a result of sporadic, postzygotic somatic pathogenic mutations. HRAS mutations have been recorded in 95% of cases, and KRAS mutations less commonly (5%).[63–65] Mosaic FGFR2-activating mutations have been reported in 2 fetuses with papillomatous, pedunculated NS, although these might represent a keratinocytic nevus syndrome.[66,67] A cerebriform subtype of NS has also been recently described due to FGFR2 mutations.[68] Given the low risk of malignant potential, practice has changed from removal to observation of the NS in most cases. Removal, if desired, ideally occurs after age 3 years given the interest in avoiding early pediatric anesthesia for elective procedures.[69–71]

NSS, also called Schimmelpenning syndrome, refers to the rare occurrence of NS, most often large or centrofacial nevi, and extracutaneous manifestations. The most frequent extracutaneous manifestation of NSS is CNS involvement, including seizures and developmental delay.[72,73] Ophthalmologic abnormalities are also common. Musculoskeletal, cardiovascular, and urogenital manifestations may occur. There can be associated endocrine abnormalities, including hypophosphatemic rickets.[74] Pathogenic variants in the RAS pathway genes (HRAS, NRAS, KRAS) have been documented.[75]

What Is New and What Is Noteworthy

- Monitor for hypophosphatemic rickets in patients with NSS.[74]
- Pathogenic mutations in NS and NSS include HRAS, KRAS and NRAS.[63–65,75]
- Mosaic FGFR2-activating mutation has been recently reported in a cerebriform subtype of NS.[68]

PHACOMATOSIS PIGMENTOKERATOTICA

The term phacomatosis pigmentokeratotica refers to the association of an organoid epidermal nevus, usually with sebaceous differentiation, and speckled lentiginous nevus (SLN).[76] The distribution of the NS usually follows Blaschko lines, whereas the SLN may be arranged in a segmental checkerboard pattern.[77] The melanocytic portion may present as a segmental tan patch in infancy and subsequently develop darker macules within the patch later in childhood. Various extracutaneous abnormalities may be present, including neurologic, ophthalmologic, and musculoskeletal, although some patients do not have extracutaneous manifestations.[78–80] PPK is considered a RASopathy with malignant potential because cutaneous and extracutaneous malignancies have been reported.[79] Sporadic pathogenic mutations in HRAS, KRAS, and BRAF have been described.[78–81] Hypophosphatemic rickets has also been noted in association with PPK.[82] Torchia and Happle[83] have recently proposed that the term phacomatosis spilosebacea replace the term PPK for select lesions.

POROKERATOTIC ADNEXAL OSTIAL NEVUS

PAON is a rare malformation classified as an eccrine hamartoma.[84] Clinically, it presents as linear hyperkeratotic papules and plaques with comedolike punctate pits and keratin plugs most commonly located on the palms or soles. Most present at birth or early childhood. Rare extracutaneous associations have included neurodevelopmental, musculoskeletal, and endocrine anomalies and idiopathic calcinosis cutis.[85,86] Hearing loss is an important feature and provides a clue to pathogenesis.[87] The GJB2 gene product is a protein called gap junction beta 2, commonly known as connexin 26. Pathogenic mutations in GBJ2/connexin 26 are found in the affected tissue of PAON as well as in keratitis ichthyosis deafness (KID) syndrome.[88–91]

What Is Noteworthy

- Pathogenic genetic changes in GBJ2/connexin 26 are found in PAON and KID syndrome.[89]
- One should be aware of the association of GBJ2/connexin 26 and hearing loss.[87]

NEVUS COMEDONICUS AND NEVUS COMEDONICUS SYNDROME

Nevus comedonicus (NC) is a rarely occurring nevus of the pilosebaceous unit; it may present as a solitary plaque or in a linear array of dilated follicular orifices plugged with keratin along Blaschko lines. The most common locations include the face, neck, or trunk.[92] Widespread and inflammatory variants may occur.[93] Histologic features of epidermolytic ichthyosis have also been noted in nevus comedonicus.[94] A somatic mutation in fibroblast growth factor receptor 2 (FGFR2), also found in Apert syndrome, a craniosynostosis syndrome associated with severe acne, was previously reported.[95] More recently, pathogenic mutations in NEK9 (never in mitosis gene A related kinase 9), which encodes a member of the family of serine/threonine protein kinases activated in cell cycle and mitosis, have been described in NC.[96,97] Nevus comedonicus syndrome (NCS) refers to the association with other abnormalities, including developmental anomalies, and extracutaneous manifestations, including skeletal and CNS abnormalities.[98,99]

What Is New

- Somatic mutations in NEK9 have been demonstrated in NC and NCS.[96–98]

BECKER NEVUS AND BECKER NEVUS SYNDROME

Becker nevus is a type of epidermal nevus that may also be referred to as Becker melanosis or pigmented hairy epidermal nevus; it most frequently presents on the trunk or proximal upper extremities as a hyperpigmented patch with irregular borders that gradually enlarges or darkens for a few years and then remains stable.[100,101] Becker nevus typically presents around puberty, although congenital cases also occur.[102] Hypertrichosis within the lesion is common but not always present. Piloerection (pseudo-Darier sign), when smooth muscle components are present in the nevus, may occur on stroking. Increased androgen receptors have been found in Becker nevi and may explain the apparent onset during puberty in many cases.[103] Although there are isolated reports of skin cancers developing within Becker nevi, they are generally not considered to have malignant potential. Laser treatment has been used to lighten the pigment as well as decrease the hypertrichosis with variable and limited long-term efficacy.[104,105]

Becker nevus syndrome refers to patients with a Becker nevus and other associated developmental defects.[106] Musculoskeletal anomalies especially of the chest wall and limb are common.[107] Somatic mutations of beta-actin (ACTB), a protein involved in the Hedgehog signaling pathway, in pilar muscles have been found in the affected tissue of patients with Becker nevi and Becker nevus syndrome as well as congenital smooth muscle hamartomas.[108–110]

What Is New

Somatic mutations of beta-actin (ACTB) in pilar muscles have been found in the affected tissue of patients with Becker nevi and Becker nevus syndrome.[108]

SUMMARY

The use of next-generation sequencing has helped to elucidate the pathogenesis of epidermal nevi and further our understanding of their systemic manifestations. When ENS is suspected, genetic evaluation plays an important role because the specific mutation may harbor clues to the associated extracutaneous manifestations and risks. The concept of germline mosaicism in association with certain nevi that may harbor more widespread pathogenic phenotypes in offspring should be considered. As more becomes known about the genetics of epidermal nevi and syndromes and testing becomes readily available, updated classification as well as targeted therapies are likely to follow.

CLINICS CARE POINTS

- Perform a full cutaneous examination for findings associates with epidermal nevi and consider specialty and genetic referral 25 appropriate.
- Recognize that targets therapies may be utilizes to manage select epidermal keratinocytic and adnexal lesions.

DISCLOSURE

The authors have no relevant conflicts of interests to disclose.

REFERENCES

1. Garcias-Ladaria J, Cuadrado Rosón M, Pascual-López M. Epidermal nevi and related syndromes – part 1: keratinocytic nevi. Actas Dermosifiliogr 2018;109(8):677–86.
2. Garcias-Ladaria J, Cuadrado Rosón M, Pascual-López M. Epidermal nevi and related syndromes – part 2: nevi derived from adnexal structures. Actas Dermosifiliogr 2018;109(8):687–98.
3. Asch S, Sugarman JL. Epidermal nevus syndromes: new insights into whorls and swirls. Pediatr Dermatol 2018;35(1):21–9.
4. Kinsler VA, Boccara O, Fraitag S, et al. Mosaic abnormalities of the skin: review and guidelines from the European Reference Network for rare skin diseases. Br J Dermatol 2020;182(3):552–63.
5. Affleck AG, Leach IH, Varma S. Two squamous cell carcinomas arising in a linear epidermal nevus in a 28-year-old female. Clin Exp Dermatol 2005;30: 382–4.
6. Horn MS, Sausker WF, Pierson DL. Basal cell epithelioma arising in a linear epidermal nevus. Arch Dermatol 1981;117:247.
7. Jeon J, Kim JH, Baek YS, et al. Eccrine poroma and eccrine porocarcinoma in linear epidermal nevus. Am J Dermatopathol 2014;36(5):430–2.

8. Hafner C, López-Knowles E, Luis NM, et al. Oncogenic PIK3Ca mutations occur in epidermal nevi and seborrheic keratoses with a characteristic mutation pattern. Proc Natl Acad Sci U S A 2007; 104(33):13450–4.

9. Hafner C, Hartmann A, Vogt T. FGFR3 mutations in epidermal nevi and seborrheic keratoses: lessons from urothelium and skin. J Invest Dermatol 2007; 127(7):1572–3.

10. Collin B, Taylor IB, Wilkie AO, et al. Fibroblast growth factor receptor 3 (FGFR3) mutation in a verrucous epidermal naevus associated with mild facial dysmorphism. Br J Dermatol 2007;156(6):1353–6.

11. Ousager LB, Bygum A, Hafner C. Identification of a novel S249C FGFR3 mutation in a keratinocytic epidermal naevus syndrome. Br J Dermatol 2012; 167(1):202–4.

12. Alkhalifah A, Fransen F, Le Duff F, et al. Laser treatment of epidermal nevi: a multicenter retrospective study with long-term follow-up. J Am Acad Dermatol 2020;83(6):1606–15.

13. Alonso-Castro L, Boixeda P, Reig I, et al. Carbon dioxide laser treatment of epidermal nevi: response and long-term follow-up. Actas Dermosifiliogr 2012;103(10):910–8.

14. Hafner C, Toll A, Gantner S, et al. Keratinocytic epidermal nevi are associated with mosaic RAS mutations. J Med Genet 2012;49(4):249–53.

15. Toll A, Fernández LC, Pons T, et al. Somatic embryonic FGFR2 mutations in keratinocytic epidermal nevi. J Invest Dermatol 2016;136(8):1718–21.

16. Dodds M, Maguiness S. Topical sirolimus therapy for epidermal nevus with features of acanthosis nigricans. Pediatr Dermatol 2019;36(4):554–5.

17. Paller AS, Syder AJ, Chan YM, et al. Genetic and clinical mosaicism in a type of epidermal nevus. N Engl J Med 1994;331(21):1408–15.

18. Mohamad J, Samuelov L, Assaf S, et al. Epidermolytic epidermal nevus caused by a somatic mutation in KRT2. Pediatr Dermatol 2021;38(2):538–40.

19. Rulo HF, van de Kerkhof PC. Treatment of inflammatory linear verrucous epidermal nevus. Dermatologica 1991;182(2):112–4.

20. Ossorio-García L, Jiménez-Gallo D, Collantes-Rodríguez C, et al. Treatment of inflammatory linear verrucous epidermal nevus pruritus with thalidomide. J Dtsch Dermatol Ges 2018;16(9):1141–2.

21. Saifaldeen RH, Fatani MI, Baltow B, et al. Successful treatment of inflammatory linear verrucous epidermal nevus with concomitant psoriasis using etanercept. Case Rep Dermatol 2018;10(1):29–34.

22. Özdemir M, Balevi A, Esen H. An inflammatory verrucous epidermal nevus concomitant with psoriasis: treatment with adalimumab. Dermatol Online J 2012;18(10):11.

23. Lee BJ, Mancini AJ, Renucci J, et al. Full-thickness surgical excision for the treatment of inflammatory linear verrucous epidermal nevus. Ann Plast Surg 2001;47:285–92.

24. Patel N, Padhiyar J, Patel A, et al. Successful amelioration of inflammatory linear verrucous epidermal nevus with topical sirolimus. Ann Dermatol 2020;32(6):534–6.

25. Barney E, Prose NS, Ramirez M. Inflammatory linear verrucous epidermal nevus treated successfully with crisaborole ointment in a 5-year-old boy. Pediatr Dermatol 2019;36(3):404–5.

26. Su WP. Histopathologic varieties of epidermal nevus. A study of 160 cases. Am J Dermatopathol 1982;4(2):161–70.

27. Sakuntabhai A, Dhitavat J, Burge S, et al. Mosaicism for ATP2A2 mutations causes segmental Darier's disease. J Invest Dermatol 2000;115(6): 1144–7.

28. Akinshemoyin Vaughn O, Hinshaw MA, Teng JM. Acantholytic dyskeratotic epidermal nevus. JAMA Dermatol 2015;151(11):1259–60.

29. Lee YI, Kim TG, Lee ST, et al. A somatic p.Phe29del mutation of connexin 26 (GJB2) manifesting as acantholytic dyskeratotic epidermal nevus. JAMA Dermatol 2019;155(5):633–5.

30. National center for biotechnology information, genetic testing registry. Tests: ATP2A2. Available at: http://www.ncbi.nlm.nih.gov/gtr/tests/516093/. Accessed May 21, 2021.

31. Konig A, Happle R, Bornholdt D, et al. Mutations in the NSDHL gene, encoding a 3beta-hydroxysteroid dehydrogenase, cause CHILD syndrome. Am J Med Genet 2000;90(4):339–46.

32. Bornholdt D, Konig A, Happle R, et al. Mutational spectrum of NSDHL in CHILD syndrome. J Med Genet 2005;42(2):e17.

33. Paller AS, van Steensel MA, Rodriguez-Martín M, et al. Pathogenesis-based therapy reverses cutaneous abnormalities in an inherited disorder of distal cholesterol metabolism. J Invest Dermatol 2011;131(11):2242–8.

34. Lai-Cheong JE, Elias PM, Paller AS. Pathogenesis-based therapies in ichthyoses. Dermatol Ther 2013;26(1):46–54.

35. Merino De Paz N, Rodriguez-Martin M, Contreras-Ferrer P, et al. Topical treatment of CHILD nevus and Sjogren-Larsson Syndrome with combined lovastatin and cholesterol. Eur J Dermatol 2011; 21(6):1026–7.

36. Biesecker L. The challenges of Proteus syndrome: diagnosis and management. Eur J Hum Genet 2006;14(11):1151–7.

37. Lindhurst MJ, Sapp JC, Teer JK, et al. A mosaic activating mutation in AKT1 associated with the Proteus syndrome. N Engl J Med 2011;365:611–9.

38. De Souza RA. Origins of the elephant man: mosaic somatic mutations cause Proteus syndrome. Clin Genet 2012;81(2):123–4.

39. Barmakian JT, Posner MA, Silver L, et al. Proteus syndrome. J Hand Surg Am 1992;17(1):32–4.

40. Keppler-Noreuil KM, Parker VE, Darling TN, et al. Somatic overgrowth disorders of the PI3K/AKT/mTOR pathway & therapeutic strategies. Am J Med Genet C Semin Med Genet 2016;172(4):402–21.

41. Cohen MM Jr. Causes of premature death in Proteus syndrome. Am J Med Genet 2001;101(1):1–3.

42. Nguyen D, Turner JT, Olsen C, et al. Cutaneous manifestations of proteus syndrome: correlations with general clinical severity. Arch Dermatol 2004;140(8):947–53.

43. Biesecker LG, Sapp JC. Proteus syndrome. In: Adam MP, Ardinger HH, Pagon RA, et al, editors. GeneReviews® [Internet]. Seattle (WA): University of Washington, Seattle; 1993–2021; 2012.

44. Keppler-Noreuil KM, Lozier J, Oden N, et al. Thrombosis risk factors in PIK3CA-related overgrowth spectrum and Proteus syndrome. Am J Med Genet C Semin Med Genet 2019;181(4):571–81.

45. Polubothu S, Al-Olabi L, Wilson L, et al. Extending the spectrum of AKT1 mosaicism: not just the Proteus syndrome. Br J Dermatol 2016;175(3):612–4.

46. Forde K, Resta N, Ranieri C, et al. Clinical experience with the AKT1 inhibitor miransertib in two children with PIK3CA-related overgrowth syndrome. Orphanet J Rare Dis 2021;16(1):109.

47. Happle R. Linear Cowden nevus: a new distinct epidermal nevus. Eur J Dermatol 2007;17(2):133–6.

48. Yehia L, Keel E, Eng C. The clinical spectrum of PTEN mutations. Annu Rev Med 2020;71:103–16.

49. Keppler-Noreuil KM, Rios JJ, Parker VE, et al. PIK3CA-related overgrowth spectrum (PROS): diagnostic and testing eligibility criteria, differential diagnosis, and evaluation. Am J Med Genet A 2015;167A(2):287–95.

50. Sapp JC, Turner JT, van de Kamp JM, et al. Newly delineated syndrome of congenital lipomatous overgrowth, vascular malformations, and epidermal nevi (CLOVE syndrome) in seven patients. Am J Med Genet A 2007;143A(24):2944–58.

51. Gucev ZS, Tasic V, Jancevska A, et al. Congenital lipomatous overgrowth, vascular malformations, and epidermal nevi (CLOVE) syndrome: CNS malformations and seizures may be a component of this disorder. Am J Med Genet A 2008;146A(20):2688–90.

52. Hughes M, Hao M, Luu M. PIK3CA vascular overgrowth syndromes: an update. Curr Opin Pediatr 2020;32(4):539–46.

53. Renatta de Grazia R, Giordano C, Cossio L, et al. CLOVES syndrome: treatment with oral Rapamycin. Report of two cases. Rev Chil Pediatr 2019;90(6):662–7.

54. Venot Q, Blanc T, Rabia SH, et al. Targeted therapy in patients with PIK3CA-related overgrowth syndrome. Nature 2018;558(7711):540–6. Erratum in: Nature. 2019;568(7752):E6.

55. Sugarman GI, Reed WB. Two unusual neurocutaneous disorders with facial cutaneous signs. Arch Neurol 1969;21:242–7.

56. Lim YH, Ovejero D, Sugarman JS, et al. Multilineage somatic activating mutations in HRAS and NRAS cause mosaic cutaneous and skeletal lesions, elevated FGF23 and hypophosphatemia. Hum Mol Genet 2014;23(2):397–407.

57. Heike CL, Cunningham ML, Steiner RD, et al. Skeletal changes in epidermal nevus syndrome: does focal bone disease harbor clues concerning pathogenesis? Am J Med Genet A 2005;139A(2):67–77.

58. Goyal A, Damle N, Kandasamy D, et al. Epidermal nevus syndrome with hypophosphatemic rickets. Indian J Endocrinol Metab 2020;24(2):227–9.

59. Aschinberg LC, Solomon LM, Zeis PM, et al. Vitamin D-resistant rickets associated with epidermal nevus syndrome: demonstration of a phosphaturic substance in the dermal lesions. J Pediatr 1977;91:56–60.

60. Athonvarangkul D, Insogna KL. New therapies for hypophosphatemia-related to FGF23 excess. Calcif Tissue Int 2021;108(1):143–57.

61. Mehregan AH, Pinkus H. Life history of organoid nevi. Special reference to nevus sebaceus of Jadassohn. Arch Dermatol 1965;91:574–88.

62. Hamilton KS, Johnson S, Smoller BR. The role of androgen receptors in the clinical course of nevus sebaceus of Jadassohn. Mod Pathol 2001;14(6):539–42.

63. Groesser L, Herschberger E, Ruetten A, et al. Postzygotic HRAS and KRAS mutations cause nevus sebaceous and Schimmelpenning syndrome. Nat Genet 2012;44(7):783–7.

64. Levinsohn JL, Tian LC, Boyden LM, et al. Whole-exome sequencing reveals somatic mutations in HRAS and KRAS, which cause nevus sebaceus. J Invest Dermatol 2013;133(3):827–30.

65. Aslam A, Salam A, Griffiths CE, et al. Naevus sebaceus: a mosaic RASopathy. Clin Exp Dermatol 2014;39(1):1–6.

66. Kuentz P, Fraitag S, Gonzales M, et al. Mosaic-activating FGFR2 mutation in two fetuses with papillomatous pedunculated sebaceous naevus. Br J Dermatol 2017;176(1):204–8.

67. Has C. Mosaicism in the skin: lumping or splitting? Br J Dermatol 2017;176(1):15–6.

68. Theiler M, Weibel L, Christen-Zaech S, et al. Cerebriform sebaceous nevus: a subtype of organoid nevus due to specific postzygotic FGFR2 mutations. J Eur Acad Dermatol Venereol 2021. https://doi.org/10.1111/jdv.17319.

69. Kamyab-Hesari K, Seirafi H, Jahan S, et al. Nevus sebaceus: a clinicopathological study of 168 cases and review of the literature. Int J Dermatol 2016; 55(2):193–200.

70. Idriss MH, Elston DM. Secondary neoplasms associated with nevus sebaceus of Jadassohn: a study of 707 cases. J Am Acad Dermatol 2014;70(2): 332–7.

71. Consensus Statement on the use of Anesthetic and sedative drugs in infants and toddlers. Smart Tots; 2015. Available at: https://smarttots.org/about/consensus-statement/. Accessed Mar 21, 2021.

72. Rizzo R, Pavone P. Nevus sebaceous and its association with neurologic involvement. Semin Pediatr Neurol 2015;22(4):302–9.

73. Kim YE, Baek ST. Neurodevelopmental aspects of RASopathies. Mol Cells 2019;42(6):441–7.

74. Narazaki R, Ihara K, Namba N, et al. Linear nevus sebaceous syndrome with hypophosphatemic rickets with elevated FGF-23. Pediatr Nephrol 2012;27(5):861–3.

75. Kuroda Y, Ohashi I, Enomoto Y, et al. A postzygotic NRAS mutation in a patient with Schimmelpenning syndrome. Am J Med Genet A 2015;167A(9): 2223–5.

76. Happle R, Hoffmann R, Restano L, et al. Phacomatosis pigmentokeratotica: a melanocytic-epidermal twin nevus syndrome. Am J Med Genet 1996;65(4): 363–5.

77. Kubo A, Yamada D. Phakomatosis Pigmentokeratotica. N Engl J Med 2019;381(15):1458.

78. Jennings L, Cummins R, Murphy GM, et al. HRAS mutation in phacomatosis pigmentokeratotica without extracutaneous disease. Clin Exp Dermatol 2017;42(7):791–2.

79. Om A, Cathey SS, Gathings RM, et al. Phacomatosis Pigmentokeratotica: a mosaic RASopathy with malignant potential. Pediatr Dermatol 2017;34(3): 352–5.

80. Martin RJ, Arefi M, Splitt M, et al. Phacomatosis pigmentokeratotica and precocious puberty associated with HRAS mutation. Br J Dermatol 2018; 178(1):289–91.

81. Kuentz P, Mignot C, St-Onge J, et al. Postzygotic BRAF p.Lys601Asn mutation in phacomatosis pigmentokeratotica with woolly hair nevus and focal cortical dysplasia. J Invest Dermatol 2016;136(5): 1060–2.

82. Bouthors J, Vantyghem MC, Manouvrier-Hanu S, et al. Phacomatosis pigmentokeratotica associated with hypophosphataemic rickets, pheochromocytoma and multiple basal cell carcinomas. Br J Dermatol 2006;155(1):225–6.

83. Torchia D, Happle R. Phacomatosis spilosebacea: a new name for a distinctive binary genodermatosis. J Am Acad Dermatol 2021.

84. Goddard DS, Rogers M, Frieden IJ, et al. Widespread porokeratotic adnexal ostial nevus: clinical features and proposal of a new name unifying porokeratotic eccrine ostial and dermal duct nevus and porokeratotic eccrine and hair follicle nevus. J Am Acad Dermatol 2009;61(6): 1060.e1-4.

85. Llamas-Velasco M, Hilty N, Kempf W. Porokeratotic adnexal ostial naevus: review on the entity and therapeutic approach. J Eur Acad Dermatol Venereol 2015;29(10):2032–7.

86. Vasudevan B, Sondhi V, Verma R, et al. A unique association of unilateral idiopathic calcinosis cutis with ipsilateral porokeratotic eccrine ostial and dermal duct nevus. Pediatr Dermatol 2015;32(1): e8–12.

87. Jamora MJ, Celis MA. Generalized porokeratotic eccrine ostial and dermal duct nevus associated with deafness. J Am Acad Dermatol 2008;59(2 Suppl 1):S43–5.

88. Easton JA, Donnelly S, Kamps MA, et al. Porokeratotic eccrine nevus may be caused by somatic connexin26 mutations. J Invest Dermatol 2012; 132(9):2184–91.

89. Lazic T, Li Q, Frank M, et al. Extending the phenotypic spectrum of keratitis-ichthyosis-deafness syndrome: report of a patient with GJB2 (G12R) Connexin 26 mutation and unusual clinical findings. Pediatr Dermatol 2012;29(3):349–57.

90. Noda K, Sugiura K, Kono M, et al. Porokeratotic eccrine ostial and dermal duct nevus with a somatic homozygous or monoallelic variant of connexin 26. J Dermatol Sci 2015;80(1):74–6.

91. Levinsohn JL, McNiff JM, Antaya RJ, et al. A Somatic p.G45E GJB2 mutation causing porokeratotic eccrine ostial and dermal duct nevus. JAMA Dermatol 2015;151(6):638–41.

92. Cestari TF, Rubim M, Valentini BC. Nevus comedonicus: case report and brief review of the literature. Pediatr Dermatol 1991;8(4):300–5.

93. Kirtak N, Inaloz HS, Karakok M, et al. Extensive inflammatory nevus comedonicus involving half of the body. Int J Dermatol 2004;43(6):434–6.

94. Zanniello R, Pilloni L, Conti B, et al. Late-onset nevus comedonicus with follicular epidermolytic hyperkeratosis-case report and review of the literature. Am J Dermatopathol 2019;41(6):453–5.

95. Munro CS, Wilkie AO. Epidermal mosaicism producing localised acne: somatic mutation in FGFR2. Lancet 1998;352(9129):704–5.

96. Levinsohn JL, Sugarman JL, Yale Center for Mendelian Genomics, McNiff JM, et al. Somatic Mutations in NEK9 Cause Nevus Comedonicus. Am J Hum Genet 2016;98(5):1030–7.

97. Juratli HA, Jägle S, Theiler M, et al. Three novel pathogenic NEK9 variants in patients with nevus

comedonicus: a case series. J Am Acad Dermatol 2021.

98. Sheppard SE, Smith A, Grand K, et al. Further delineation of the phenotypic spectrum of nevus comedonicus syndrome to include congenital pulmonary airway malformation of the lung and aneurysm. Am J Med Genet A 2020;182(4):746–54.

99. Torchia D. Nevus comedonicus syndrome: a systematic review of the literature. Pediatr Dermatol 2021;38(2):359–63.

100. Ballone E, Fazii P, Lappa G, et al. Prevalence of Becker's nevi in a population of young men in central Italy. J Am Acad Dermatol 2003;48(5):795.

101. Patrizi A, Medri M, Raone B, et al. Clinical characteristics of Becker's nevus in children: report of 118 cases from Italy. Pediatr Dermatol 2012;29(5):571–4.

102. Sood A, D'Souza P, Verma KK. Becker's naevus occurring at birth and in early childhood. Acta Derm Venereol 1998;78(4):311.

103. Grande Sarpa H, Harris R, Hansen CD, et al. Androgen receptor expression patterns in Becker's nevi: an immunohistochemical study. J Am Acad Dermatol 2008;59(5):834–8.

104. Momen S, Mallipeddi R, Al-Niaimi F. The use of lasers in Becker's naevus: an evidence-based review. J Cosmet Laser Ther 2016;18(4):188–92.

105. Zhong Y, Yang B, Huang L, et al. Lasers for Becker's nevus. Lasers Med Sci 2019;34(6):1071–9.

106. Happle R, Koopman RJ. Becker nevus syndrome. Am J Med Genet 1997;68:357–61.

107. Danarti R, König A, Salhi A, et al. Becker's nevus syndrome revisited. J Am Acad Dermatol 2004;51(6):965–9.

108. Torchia D. Becker nevus syndrome: a 2020 update. J Am Acad Dermatol 2021. https://doi.org/10.1016/j.jaad.2021.03.095.

109. Cai ED, Sun BK, Chiang A, et al. Postzygotic mutations in beta-actin are associated with Becker's nevus and Becker's nevus syndrome. J Invest Dermatol 2017;137(8):1795.

110. Atzmony L, Ugwu N, Zaki TD, et al. Post-zygotic ACTB mutations underlie congenital smooth muscle hamartomas. J Cutan Pathol 2020;47(8):681–5.

Normal Skin Findings and Cultural Practices in Pediatric Patients with Skin of Color

Nnenna G. Agim, MD[a],*, Alexandra J. Morquette, BA[b],
Candrice R. Heath, MD[c]

KEYWORDS

- Skin of color • Pediatric dermatology • Cultural practices • Hair

KEY POINTS

- Awareness of normal skin findings in skin of color informs calibration of clinical presentations, allowing reassurance where appropriate.
- Understanding the unique functions of ethnic skin phenotypes can influence proper selection of over the counter and prescribed products, allowing family-physician care consensus.
- Inquiry into traditional grooming practices can modify assessment of skin and hair findings in patients with skin of color, reducing concern for alternate grave diagnoses.

INTRODUCTION

The understanding of melanocytes is fundamental to the study of dermatology. This dendritic cell underlies the most feared primary cutaneous malignancy, fuels escalating progress in immunotherapy strategies, and invariably underlies entire socioeconomic constructs consciously or unconsciously based on skin tone. One cell type produces and packages varying combinations of eumelanin and pheomelanin in distinctive melanosomes for transport to keratinocytes in the epidermis, hair shafts, irises, gingivae, nail matrices, and cochlea. Beyond diffuse distribution, melanocytes congregate in nevi and increase melanin production upon UV induction in ephelides or following inflammation, the latter more prominently in darker skin types. Globally, skin of color predominates, occurring in greater than 75% of the human population.[1] According to United States national census data, the estimated combined proportion of people identifying as black, Hispanic, or a combination thereof is reported as 39.9%.[2] People with skin of color who do not acknowledge these identifying categories are not captured in this data. As such, an understanding of normal variations in pigmentation between and within ethno-genotypes can enhance a physician's interpretation of aberrancy or disease, when present. The same knowledge base also equips the practitioner to provide reassurance when appropriate. Just as skin tones vary, so do cultural practices. These practices may have an impact on diagnosis, presentation, or treatment of diseases in those with skin of color.

NORMAL SKIN FINDINGS
Biology of Skin of Color

Melanocytes appear in human fetal skin at approximately week 8 of gestation following migration from the neural crest. There they populate both suprabasal and basal layers of the nascent epidermis. Visible melanin production begins between weeks 12 and 16, with transfer estimated to occur from week 20 through the postnatal

[a] University of Texas Southwestern, Dallas, TX, USA; [b] Lewis Katz School of Medicine, Temple University, 3500 North Broad Street, Philadelphia, PA 19140, USA; [c] Lewis Katz School of Medicine, Temple University, 3401 North Broad Street, 5-OPB Dermatology, Philadelphia, PA 19140, USA
* Corresponding author. 2350 North Stemmons Freeway, Dallas, TX 75220.
E-mail addresses: Nnenna.Agim@childrens.com; NGAGIM@childrens.com

Dermatol Clin 40 (2022) 73–81
https://doi.org/10.1016/j.det.2021.09.001

period.[3] The evolution of melanogenesis during the perinatal period is more apparent in children with darker skin tones. When melanocyte precursors fail to migrate, proliferate, or produce adequate/functional amounts of melanin, a variety of congenital syndromes may ensue, such as albinism, piebaldism and Waardenburg syndrome, where skin, hair, and/or irises are affected.

In all skin types, 1 melanocyte interacts via dendrites with approximately 36 keratinocytes, forming a melanocyte-keratinocyte unit. Melanosomes produce varying ratios of brown eumelanin and pheomelanin, which varies from yellow to red in color. A person's unique composition of these melanins and their dispersion within the epidermal layers determines their visible complexion. In darker skin, the melanosomes are more productive, larger, dispersed singly or in smaller groups, and sustain their contents for more prolonged periods compared with lighter skin tones. They also are present in most layers of the epidermis, compared with basal confinement in white skin.[1]

Melanocytes increase production of the genetically determined eumelanin/pheomelanin ratios, rather than their absolute number, from birth through infancy, accounting for the evolution of skin appearance in newborns during the first few months of life. This progression of skin darkening from infancy over the first few months of life is more evident in children with skin of color.[1]

Several studies seeking to describe differences in skin function based on ethnicity have investigated transepidermal water loss, water content, stratum corneum thickness, corneocyte surface area, and skin pH, with mixed and controversial results. These studies report conflicting results for each ethnic skin type given variance in methods of measurement, body sites tested, and state of the skin when studied (pretreated occluded skin yielding different results from untreated skin). Most of these studies are in adult patients; therefore, extrapolation to the pediatric population is speculative. The dermoepidermal junction thickness, melanophage size/number, collagen fiber fragments, fibroblast size, and number have been reported as increased in darker skin, along with increased compaction of the dermis.[1] Vitamin D levels have been implicated in several systemic and cutaneous disorders and notably are lower in darker skin.[1]

Hair is a renewable organ that can be modified with minimal consequence. Hair follicles begin development after 60 days of gestation on the face, developing on the rest of the body by the fifth month. Vellus hairs replace lanugo hairs (the latter more common in prematurity) and may be seen in term births, in all areas except the scalp, where terminal hairs predominate.[4] Melanocytes within the bulge produce the melanin variants transferred to the hair shaft, creating visible hair color. There is little variation in darker hair color types where eumelanin predominates. With increasing ratios of pheomelanin, variation may occur during transition from infancy to older ages and based on environmental factors, such as sun exposure.

A variety of methods have been proposed to categorize hair texture. The classic oversimplified method of comparison discusses hair types as white, Asian, or African, based on cross-sectional and cuticular characteristics. Compared with white hair shafts, which are round or symmetrically elliptical in section, African heritage hair types have a larger-diameter, flattened, elliptical appearance and show asymmetric inner root sheaths. A golf club–shaped bulb and paired grouping of follicles have been noted as distinctive dermatopathologic findings in African American hair by Miteva and Tosti.[5] Asian hair types have been described as circular on cross-section, yielding straight, cylindrical hair shafts.[6] Curvature or spiraling of the hair follicle itself also has been reported in African American hair.[7] In 2007, a consortium of dermatologists sought to reclassify hair texture objectively, regardless of geographic origin, by employing a scoring system based on assessment of wave crests along a specified length (6 cm), curve diameter of hair shafts, and the tightness of a hair shaft coil within a predetermined 0.98-cm diameter circle. A series of 8 hair types thereby were ascertained, and, as expected, certain qualities converge along genotypic and geographic backgrounds, however, with a broader range of expression, better accounting for global diversity.[8] Type VIII hair for example, reportedly is absent in white, Brazilian, and Asian study participants but increasingly represented in African American, Caribbean, and African diaspora heritage patients.

Hair texture may be relevant in disease, for example, styling products used to modify hair deemed coarse result in specific complications, compared with those used for routine grooming of hair with finer texture. Scalp burns can be caused by hair relaxers; contact dermatitis can result from multi-ingredient ointment-based hair conditioners. Increased water loss from the cuticle in more tightly coiled hairs creates dryness, necessitating use of products acting as humectants. These typically take the form of styling oils or pomades. Occlusion of follicular ostia upon application to adjacent skin may result in acneiform eruptions. Contact dermatitis also is an important consideration, depending on the composition of these hair care products. Some investigators have postulated that use of oils and pomades hampers evaluation of the scale in tinea capitis.[9]

Because tightly coiled hair is not partitioned easily, deliberate hands-on assessment by an examiner with cultural humility[10] affords better visualization for scale. A swab for fungal culture of potentially involved areas is important, especially when tinea capitis is a diagnostic consideration.

The asymmetric diameter along the coiled hair shaft fosters uneven distribution of sebum, a natural moisturizer, enhancing dryness and thus fragility.[11] This natural tendency increases risk for hair damage from styling practices, which employ mechanical stress on the hair shafts. The slower distribution of sebum along the coiled hair shaft however allows less frequent washing.[6] Traction alopecia and acquired trichorrhexis nodosa are 2 common examples of styling-related hair disorders found in African, African American, and Afro-Caribbean hair types. When hair is styled with heat, chemical dyes, chemical straighteners, and similar tools, the cuticle is damaged, exposing cortical fibers. These processes compound the natural fragility of tightly coiled hair. Keratin filaments contain cysteine, which can cross-link to form disulfide bonds. These bonds contribute to the curl pattern of hair shafts more strongly that van der Waals forces, which, although also present, can be severed by simple exposure to water.[12] Many of the aforementioned styling tools and practices are aimed at breaking the disulfide bonds, reversion of which directly affects frequency of their employment. An understanding of hair care practices based on the biology discussed is essential for the dermatologist because the implications may extend beyond cutaneous disease. A survey of more than 100 adult patients with skin of color revealed that greater than 40% of respondents spend more than 60 minutes on their hair styles weekly, and many reported forfeiting physical activity to protect their hair. Given ongoing concern for the rise in pediatric obesity, whether isolated or in the context of disease, any hindrance to physical activity may pose health risks. Thus, hair care and styling in patients with skin of color may play a unique role in their overall health and should be assessed in culturally sensitive ways.

CLINICAL OBSERVATIONS BASED ON BIOLOGY: BENIGN, NORMAL FINDINGS
Newborn Skin Tone

As described in the introduction, infants with darker skin tones show an evolution of their skin tone from infancy through early childhood. Their overall skin color at birth may be much lighter than their final complexion because melanocyte migration, melanosome production, and melanin transfer, which began in utero, actively evolve postpartum. Deeper

pigmentation of the scrotal and labial areas is common; 1 study of more than 1700 Asian male infants demonstrated this feature in one-third of the cohort.[13] Most families are aware of the color change phenomenon, and inspection of the auricles and interphalangeal joints may offer a preview of their expected skin tone.

Congenital Hypertrichosis

Universal hypertrichosis, which presents with normally pigmented abundant hair involving the back, buttocks, preauricular area, and proximal extremities, is considered a normal variant in South Asian, Hispanic, and Mediterranean ethnicities.[14] The hair density may decrease spontaneously in density over time. Pathologic congenital hypertrichosis may follow intrauterine exposure to high-dose corticosteroids, diethylstilbestrol, or minoxidil. Subcategories include hypertrichosis universalis and congenital hypertrichosis lanuginose, where the long hair is lighter colored and accompanied by dental anomalies.

Futcher Lines

Futcher lines, as described in **Table 1**, are reproducible patterns of dorsoventral pigmentary demarcation most apparent in darker skin types beginning at approximately age 6 months. Also termed Voigt lines, given a description in the 1800s by an Austrian anatomist, they are thought to represent gradients of melanin production following melanocyte migration patterns initiated during embryogenesis.[15] This benign pigmentary variation requires no intervention other than recognition. Alexandrite laser has been employed for treatment in a single case; however, this is not necessary.[16] These lines (especially group B) may be enhanced more during pregnancy and show a predilection for female patients; dermoscopy can confirm the presence of increase melanin deposition in darker areas.[17] Facial involvement should be distinguished from melasma in adults.[18]

Oral Pigmentation

Gingival pigmentation usually is physiologic in darker skin types and overall benign. It results from genetically determined quantities of melanin deposition in the basal and suprabasal mucosal epithelia with labial predominance. Incidence increases with age and no treatment is necessary. The differential diagnosis includes pigmentation from medications, Addison disease, Peutz-Jeghers syndrome, lichen planus, and postinflammatory changes associated with dental procedures or orthodontics.[19]

Lingual melanosis describes melanin deposition in and around lingual papillae in a circumscribed

Table 1
Pigmentary demarcation lines

Pigmentary Demarcation Line Groups	Anatomic Location
A	Upper extremities extending to the chest
B	Lower extremities
C	Midchest to midabdomen
D	Paraspinal posterior midline
E	Bilateral chest; clavicle to areolae
F	Between temple and malar cheek, V-shaped
G	Between temple and malar cheek, W-shaped
H	Lower facial, from perioral area to chin

fashion. These lesions usually are present from birth, may be single or multiple, and do not favor a particular location on the tongue.[20] The macules are deep brown or black and may enlarge as the child grows. Black hairy tongue and oral melanoma are exceedingly rare in pediatric patients but may be considered in patients with iatrogenic or congenital immunosuppression for the former or with exophytic, symptomatic, asymmetric presentation, and/or rapid expansion for the latter. Incidence may be increased in darker skin types. Appearance in adulthood also has been reported; in this population, smoking history should be ascertained and malignancy excluded.[21] There are few reported cases of malignant degeneration in adults, so clinical monitoring is recommended.[22]

Nails

Longitudinal melanonychia occurs with greater frequency in patients with skin of color. Involvement of multiple fingernails and/or toenails is a reassuring sign of benignity and often a sign of physiologic activation of quiescent nail bed melanocytes, for example, from trauma, such as sports. For patients with involvement of a single nail, close assessment for potentially worrisome characteristics, such as rapid or aggressive growth or advancement beyond the nail, should be conducted on a regular basis.[23] No specific therapy is required for benign nail pigmentation. Rapid onset or diffuse involvement in the context of systemic signs and symptoms should prompt further assessment for Addison disease or Cronkhite-Canada syndrome if suspected. Addison disease and Cronkhite-Canada syndrome may present with diffuse cutaneous hyperpigmentation and abdominal pain, in the latter condition due to underlying gastrointestinal polyps. Laugier–Hunziker syndrome is pigmentation that

may affect the lips, oral mucosa, and acral surfaces as well as the nail due to melanosis without melanocytosis.[24] Some commonly used dermatologic medications, such as tetracyclines, also can cause nail pigmentation; given systemic administration of the drug, multiple nails are affected.

CULTURAL PRACTICES THAT MAY BE RELEVANT IN PEDIATRIC PATIENTS WITH SKIN OF COLOR

The cultural practices explored herein highlight traditional, current, and past practices. It is recognized that all people with shared heritage do not adhere to the exact same traditional or common practices. These examples serve as historical references of cultural practices. Familiarity with the findings and their potential basis can improve cultural sensitivity when assessing pediatric patients from diverse ethnic backgrounds.

African Descent

Hair grease/oil

Population: African descent
Cultural practice: application of grease and oil to scalp
Cultural belief: to help moisturize the hair or scalp; helps hair to grow. A 2011 study examining common hair care practices in African American girls found that 99% of girls included in the study used oil, grease, or lotion on their hair or scalp.[25]
Implication for pediatric patients with skin of color: application of oils and grease to the scalp may cause a delay in recognition of scaly scalp conditions like seborrheic dermatitis-like variant of tinea capitis or seborrheic dermatitis and pomade acne in black children.[25,26]

Braids, twists, and extensions

Population: African descent

Cultural practice: hairstyles with braids, twists, or extensions

Cultural belief: display of cultural expression and beauty with the ability to create intricate designs and patterns, thought to be protective styling of the hair

Implication for pediatric patients with skin of color: these styles may be damaging rather than protective to hair, because they can cause excessive traction on the scalp due to the tightness of the style or weight that the hair extensions place on the hair shaft. African children who use these styles are more likely to be affected by traction alopecia and central centrifugal cicatricial alopecia.[25,27] These styles not only may put children at risk of developing these conditions but also may pose a challenge in diagnosis. There may be less access to certain areas of the scalp. Acne keloidalis nuchae has been associated with boys who have their hair repeatedly cut close to the scalp and nape of the neck.[27] Longer hair styles are protective against this condition; however, when assessing patients with longer styles, inspecting the entire scalp margin should not be neglected, because these may be cropped close and camouflaged by natural hair or extensions.

Relaxers

Population: African descent

Cultural practice: use of alkaline chemical hair relaxers, more commonly used in girls than boys; permanently straightens tightly coiled hair

Cultural belief: straighten hair for ease of handling and styling

Implication for pediatric patients with skin of color: there is risk of chemical burning of the scalp and skin and of hair breakage when applied incorrectly. A Nigerian study found that repeated relaxer use had an increased association with scarring alopecia compared with those who did not use relaxer.[28] A South African study found that girls with relaxed hair developed traction alopecia more frequently, possibly due to the increased fragility of the hair, leaving it less resistant to traction.[27] A similar risk to the hair and scalp exists with repeated heat application, commonly with hot combs or flat irons in children. One study found that the common initiation of heat and chemical relaxer use in girls' hair was between ages 4 years and 6 years of age and between ages 4 years and 8 years of age, respectively.[25]

Body markings

Population: African descent

Cultural practice: patterned body markings with burning, cutting, and scarring of the skin

Cultural belief: decorative purposes and tribal identification; also for medicinal purposes[29]

Implication for pediatric patients with skin of color: scarring and body markings may lead to keloids. Body markings with burning, cutting, and scarring of the skin in children may be mistaken for child abuse in countries unfamiliar with this practice. Hence, recognition may be important in immigrant populations.

Female genital mutilation

Population: Western, Eastern, and Northeastern African countries; some in the Middle East and Asia

Cultural practice: female genital mutilation/circumcision in adolescent girls involves cutting and removal of external genitalia.

Cultural belief: female genital mutilation done for religious reasons; done to preserve virginity, reduce sexual pleasure, and increase likelihood of marriage; or considered a rite of passage[30]

Implication for pediatric patients with skin of color: female genital mutilation has no medical benefit and poses significant morbidity and mortality.[30] Long-term complications include urinary and vaginal problems, problems with sexual intercourse, increased risk of childbirth complications, and psychological problems, such as depression and anxiety.[30] More than 3 million girls are at risk annually.[30]

Latinx/Hispanic

Chili Peppers

Population: Mexican

Cultural practice: use of chili peppers

Cultural belief: chili peppers are a spice used commonly in Mexican cuisine.

Implication for pediatric patients with skin of color: capsaicin dermatitis occurs due to the handling of chili peppers. Food handlers and cooks are at increased risk.[26,31] Parents who handle chili peppers can transfer the irritative substances to their children's skin causing capsaicin dermatitis.

Pomades and greases

Population: Latinx

Cultural practice: use of pomades and grease in the hair

Cultural belief: used to moisturize hair and also for stylistic purposes. One example, decades ago, was the pachuco style of adolescents in the 1940s, using pomades to slick hair back.

Implication for pediatric patients with skin of color: potentially comedogenic pomades and oils increase the risk of pomade acne on the forehead, face, and neck.[31]

Circumcision

Population: Latino boys

Cultural practice: circumcision

Cultural belief: approximately fewer than 20% of male babies are circumcised in Mexico, Central America, and South America.[32] Circumcision is performed in infants for cultural, religious, and hygienic reasons.

Implication for pediatric patients with skin of color: balanitis xerotica obliterans (BXO), or penile lichen sclerosus, has a high prevalence in male Latinos and may be related to lack of circumcision.[31] A 2005 study suspects that the incidence of childhood BXO is higher than assumed previously and also was a cause of secondary phimosis in boys.[33–35] In most cases, circumcision is curative for penile lichen sclerosus.

Asian

Coining

Population: East Asian

Cultural practice: coining—the practice entails applying hot oils on the skin, and firmly stroking and scraping the skin, traditionally with the edge of a coin. Other objects, such as spoons (spooning), jar lids, and combs, also have been used.[36]

Cultural belief: coining is thought to reduce fever, headache, and flu symptoms.

Implication for pediatric patients with skin of color: dermatologic effects of this practice include ecchymotic streaks and burns in the direction of the strokes, often forming a pine tree distribution.[36,37] These cutaneous findings could be mistaken for child abuse.[38]

Cupping

Population: Asian but also is performed by people in the Middle East, Latin America, and Eastern Europe

Cultural practice: cupping involves the use of a heated cup placed on the skin. As the cup cools, it creates a vacuum that pulls the underlying skin into the cup. Cups traditionally are glass, but bamboo or alternate materials have been used.[39] There are many kinds of cupping, including wet, moving, flash, retained, and needle cupping.[40]

Cultural belief: it is thought to improve circulation, draw out toxins, improve back pain and muscle aches, and treat acne.[36]

Implication for pediatric patients with skin of color: cupping can cause erythematous streaks with moving cups, epithelial cell injury, and vascular abrasions, leading to ecchymoses, and purpura, which can be mistaken for vasculitis, other dermatoses, and child abuse.[41]

Moxibustion

Population: Asian

Cultural practice: moxibustion is a traditional Asian practice that involves the ignition and burning of moxa herb over the skin. This burning herb either is blown out before it touches the skin or allowed to linger until the skin turns red or is burned.

Cultural belief: moxibustion is used to treat asthma,[26] pain,[26] and atopic dermatitis[26,36] in Asian cultures. In combination with acupuncture, there have been studies of moxibustion's use in other diseases affecting children, such as cerebral palsy,[42] myopia,[43] and neurogenic frequent micturition.[44]

Implication for pediatric patients with skin of color: burning of the skin from moxibustion not only can lead to burns and scars but also may be mistaken for child abuse. It is important to have cultural competence when evaluating pediatric patients who may have lesions pertaining to these practices.

Henna

Population: South Asian, Indian, Middle Eastern, and some African populations

Cultural practice: application of henna to the skin. Henna is derived from the leaves of the henna plant, and crushed into a paste.

Cultural belief: henna is considered a cooling agent for the skin; used for sun protection, dying skin and hair, and decoration. Henna tattoos are an integral cultural practice of Indian celebrations, such as weddings and holidays. Adult women, adolescents, and children may participate.

Implication for pediatric patients with skin of color: allergic contact dermatitis may occur in children with sensitization to para-phenylenediamine, an additive that is used in modern henna formulations, also known as black henna.[45,46] Henna is a reddish-brown color, and para-phenylenediamine is added to turn the color black. Allergic contact dermatitis may result in postinflammatory hyperpigmentation in the pattern of where the henna as initially was applied.

American Indian

Botanicals and plants

Population: traditional Native American

Cultural practice: use of plants and natural botanicals. The yerba santa plant (*Eriodictyon californicum*) is indigenous to California and has been used for centuries by the Amah Mutsun tribe. *E parryi* or poodle-dog shrub is a close relative also native to California.

Cultural belief: yerba santa leaves are used in products that moisturize the skin[47] and to treat many ailments, including headaches, when placed directly on the forehead,[48] and acute bronchitis.[49] *E parryi* is used medicinally for the treatment of rheumatism.

Implication for pediatric patients with skin of color: no specific skin condition has yet been identified with the use of yerba santa. *E parryi* is considered a severe skin irritant and has been linked to cases of allergic contact dermatitis.[50]

Sacred hair and nails

Population: traditional Native American

Cultural practice: hair styling and management

Cultural belief: certain styles signify band or tribe identity.[51] Hair has a connection to spirituality. In the Navajo tradition, it is taboo to cut a baby's hair when they are small, because this may interfere with their intelligence as they grow. It is ritualistic for expectant mothers to loosen their hair and refrain from placing it in a braid or knot while laboring.[52] A study that aimed to gain insight into the use of biological samples for research purposes in Native American communities found that they were much more reluctant to give samples of hair and nail clippings compared with urine or blood samples.[53] Hair and nail sampling was considered more invasive than drawing blood or collecting urine.

Implication for pediatric patients with skin of color: it is important to keep the sacred nature of hair and nails in mind when evaluating Native American patients who are adherent to traditional cultural practices, particularly when performing physical examinations and procedures that may involve touching, moving, or cutting the hair and nails.

Inuit

Inuit women tattoos

Population: Inuit women of Alaska and Canada

Cultural practice: facial and body tattooing. The needles used to create tattoos traditionally are made of bone or whale sinew.

Cultural belief: In the nineteenth and twentieth centuries, this spiritual tradition was banned by missionaries. Its resurgence has occurred recently, in an attempt to preserve the tradition and reclaim its honor and beauty.[54,55] Each marking signifies a special moment in their life or an accomplishment. Stripes on the chin can be found in adolescents that can signify their first period, and a "V" on the forehead signifies entering womanhood.[55]

Implication for pediatric patients with skin of color: in most states, tattooing of a minor without parental consent is unlawful, so it is important to ask questions and be aware of cultural traditions when seeing tattoo markings on pediatric patients.

Native Hawaiian/Pacific Islander

Tā moko

Population: Māori people of Eastern Polynesia

Cultural practice: called *tā moko*, this tattooing practice involves carving the skin with an *uhi*, or chisel made of bone, leaving grooves and indentations in the skin, and then pigmenting with burnt wood or *āwheto* (*Ophiocordyceps robertsii*), a fungus native to New Zealand. More modern versions use needle tattooing.

Cultural belief: used as a rite of passage in young Māori people of Eastern Polynesia going through puberty, signifying their transition from childhood to adulthood. The tattooed symbols can be used to demonstrate status and rank of individuals in their community. Today, tā moko is performed as a sign of cultural identity and appreciation of the Māori language and culture.[56]

Implication for pediatric patients with skin of color: similar to the tattooing of Inuit women; a physician's awareness of tā moko as a cultural practice supervised by parents is important.

SUMMARY

Globally, skin of color is the predominant human phenotype, although distribution varies geographically. Various ethno-genotypes combine with increasing frequency over time, increasing the diversity of skin types that may present with dermatologic diagnoses. Understanding the biology of a variety of skin tones and ethnic practices congruent with distribution of skin tone is invaluable to any physician who wishes to practice culturally competent, expert skin care. Pediatric patients should be approached with sensitivity and humble inquiry, especially when cultural practices unbeknownst to the provider might inform the etiology of altered skin, hair, and nails.

CLINICS CARE POINTS

- An awareness of normal skin findings in patients with skin of color can prevent unusual alarm or cause for worry.
- Familiarity with possible traditional skin and hair care practices associated with skin of color ethnic groups can inform features present on physical exam and improve recommendations for personal care and prescribed products.

DISCLOSURE

N.G. Agim, A.J. Morquette, and C.R. Heath—nothing to disclose.

REFERENCES

1. Adegbenro A, Taylor S. Structural, physiological, functional, and cultural differences in skin of color. In: Alexis AF, Barbosa VH, editors. Skin of color: a practical guide to dermatologic diagnosis and treatment. New York: Springer; 2013. p. 1–19.
2. US Census Bureau. Race and Ethnicity. 2019. Available at: https://data.census.gov/cedsci/profile?q=United+States&g=0100000US.
3. Eichenfield LF, Frieden IJ, Mathes EF, et al. Fetal skin development. Neonatal and infant dermatology. 3rd edition. Elsevier Saunders; 2015. p. 5. chap 1.
4. Eichenfield LF, Frieden IJ, Mathes EF, et al. Structure and function of newborn skin. Neonatal and infant dermatology. 3rd edition. Elsevier Saunders; 2015. p. 18–9. chap 2.
5. Miteva M, Tosti A'. A detective look' at hair biopsies from African-American patients. Br J Dermatol 2012; 166(6):1289–94.
6. Diana Draelos Z. The biology of hair care. Dermatol Clin 2000;18(4):651–8.
7. McMichael A, Callender V. Hair and scalp disorders in pigmented skins. In: Halder R, editor. Dermatology and dermatological therapy of pigmented skins. Boca Raton, Florida: CRC Press; 2005. p. 63–4. chap 4.
8. Loussouarn G, Garcel AL, Lozano I, et al. Worldwide diversity of hair curliness: a new method of assessment. Int J Dermatol 2007;46(Suppl 1):2–6.
9. Paller A, Mancini A. An overview of dermatologic diagnosis. Hurwitz clinical pediatric dermatology. 4th edition. Elsevier Health Sciences; 2011. p. 8. chap 1.
10. Grayson C, Heath C. An approach to examining tightly coiled hair among patients with hair loss in race-discordant patient-physician interactions. JAMA Dermatol 2021. https://doi.org/10.1001/jamadermatol.2021.0338.
11. Haskin A, Kwatra SG, Aguh C. Breaking the cycle of hair breakage: pearls for the management of acquired trichorrhexis nodosa. J Dermatolog Treat 2017;28(4):322–6.
12. Bolduc C, Shapiro J. Hair care products: waving, straightening, conditioning, and coloring. Clin Dermatol 2001;19(4):431–6.
13. Tsai FJ, Tsai CH. Birthmarks and congenital skin lesions in Chinese newborns. J Formos Med Assoc 1993;92(9):838–41.
14. Saleh D, Yarrarapu SNS, Cook C. Hypertrichosis. 2021 Jul 23. In: StatPearls [Internet]. Treasure Island (FL): StatPearls Publishing; 2021.
15. Ł Zieleniewski, Schwartz RA, Goldberg DJ, et al. Voigt-Futcher pigmentary demarcation lines. J Cosmet Dermatol 2019;18(3):700–2.
16. Bukhari IA. Effective treatment of Futcher's lines with Q-switched alexandrite laser. J Cosmet Dermatol 2005;4(1):27–8.
17. Russo F, Flori ML, Taddeucci P, et al. Pigmentary demarcation lines of Voigt-Futcher: Dermoscopic and reflectance confocal microscopy features. Skin Res Technol 2020;26(3):440–2.
18. Al-Samary A, Al Mohizea S, Bin-Saif G, et al. Pigmentary demarcation lines on the face in Saudi women. Indian J Dermatol Venereol Leprol 2010; 76(4):378–81.
19. Rosebush MS, Briody AN, Cordell KG. Black and brown: non-neoplastic pigmentation of the oral mucosa. Head Neck Pathol 2019;13(1):47–55.
20. Chaput L, Samimi M, Maruani A. Congenital melanotic macules of the tongue. J Pediatr 2016;174: 270. https://doi.org/10.1016/j.jpeds.2016.03.054.
21. Suzuki HS, Souza TBC, Werner B. Lingual melanotic macule - the first case report in an adult patient. An Bras Dermatol 2018;93(2):310–1.
22. Kaehler KC, Russo PA, Egberts F, et al. Metastatic melanoma of the tongue arising from oral melanosis. Arch Dermatol 2008;144(4):558–60.
23. Burleigh A, Lam JM. Pediatric longitudinal melanonychia. CMAJ 2017;189(34):E1093.
24. Moore RT, Chae KA, Rhodes AR. Laugier and Hunziker pigmentation: a lentiginous proliferation of melanocytes. J Am Acad Dermatol 2004;50(5 Suppl):S70–4.

25. Rucker Wright D, Gathers R, Kapke A, et al. Hair care practices and their association with scalp and hair disorders in African American girls. J Am Acad Dermatol 2011;64(2):253–62.

26. Halder RM. Dermatological disorders and cultural practices. Dermatologist 2002;10(8).

27. Khumalo NP, Jessop S, Gumedze F, et al. Hairdressing is associated with scalp disease in African schoolchildren. Br J Dermatol 2007;157(1):106–10.

28. Nnoruka EN. Hair loss: is there a relationship with hair care practices in Nigeria? Int J Dermatol 2005;44(Suppl 1):13–7. Erratum in: Int J Dermatol. 2006 Jan;45(1):92. Nnoruka, Nkechi Edith [corrected to Nnoruka, Edith Nkechi]. PMID: 16187950.

29. Arfan-ul-Bari, Khan MB. Dermatological disorders related to cultural practices in black Africans of Sierra Leone. J Coll Physicians Surg Pak 2007;17(5):249–52. PMID: 17553318.

30. World Health Organization. Female genital mutilation. 2018. Available at: https://www.who.int/newsroom/fact-sheets/detail/female-genital-mutilation. Accessed April 16, 2021.

31. Moore MM, Sanchez M. Dermatological disease in Latinos in the USA. Expert Rev Dermatol 2007;2(1):87–100.

32. Circumcision Male. Global trends and determinants of prevalence, safety and acceptability. Geneva: World Health Organization; 2008.

33. Kiss A, Király L, Kutasy B, et al. High incidence of Balanitis Xerotica Obliterans in boys with Phimosis. Pediatr Dermatol 2005;22(4):305–8.

34. Eisenberg ML, Galusha D, Kennedy WA, et al. The relationship between neonatal circumcision, urinary tract infection, and health. World J Mens Health 2018;36(3):176–82.

35. Goodman MT, Hernandez BY, Shvetsov YB. Demographic and pathologic differences in the incidence of invasive penile cancer in the United States, 1995-2003. Cancer Epidemiol Biomarkers Prev 2007;16(9):1833–9.

36. Lilly E, Kundu RV. Dermatoses secondary to Asian cultural practices. Int J Dermatol 2012;51(4):372–9. quiz 379-82.

37. Ponder A, Lehman LB. 'Coining' and 'coning': an unusual complication of unconventional medicine. Neurology 1994;44(4):774–5.

38. Tan A, Mallika P. Coining: an ancient treatment widely practiced among asians. Malays Fam Physician 2011;6(2–3):97–8. PMID: 25606235; PMCID: PMC4170418.

39. Vashi NA, Patzelt N, Wirya S, et al. Dermatoses caused by cultural practices: Therapeutic cultural practices. J Am Acad Dermatol 2018;79(1):1–16.

40. Mehta P, Dhapte V. Cupping therapy: a prudent remedy for a plethora of medical ailments. J Tradit Complement Med 2015;5(3):127–34.

41. Killion CM. Cultural healing practices that mimic child abuse. Ann Forensic Res Anal 2017;4(2):1042.

42. Tang Y, Cao Z, Xia Y, et al. Effectiveness and safety of pure acupuncture and moxibustion in the treatment of children with cerebral palsy: A protocol for systematic review and meta analysis. Medicine (Baltimore) 2021;100(4):e23907. https://doi.org/10.1097/MD.0000000000023907. PMID: 33530188; PMCID: PMC7850675.

43. Shang X, Chen L, Litscher G, et al. Acupuncture and lifestyle myopia in primary school children-results from a transcontinental pilot study performed in comparison to moxibustion. Medicines (Basel) 2018;5(3):95.

44. Xie S-l, Liao X-y. Suspended moxibustion plus point injection for 56 children with neurogenic frequent micturition. J Acupuncture Tuina Sci 2010;8(4):238–9.

45. Lim SP, Prais L, Foulds IS. Henna tattoos for children: a potential source of para-phenylenediamine and thiuram sensitization. Br J Dermatol 2004;151(6):1271.

46. de Groot AC. Side-effects of henna and semi-permanent 'black henna' tattoos: a full review. Contact Dermatitis 2013;69(1):1–25.

47. Juliano C, Magrini GA. Cosmetic functional ingredients from botanical sources for anti-pollution skincare products. Cosmetics 2018;5(1):19.

48. Anderson MK. YERBA SANTA, A medicinal plant extraordinaire. Amah Mutsun Tribal Band. Available at: http://amahmutsun.org/land-trust-newsevents/yerba-santa-a-medicinal-plant-extraordinaire. Accessed April 10, 2021.

49. Stuver E. Yerba Santa and Grindelia Robusta in acute bronchitis. Med News 1885. 1882-1905.

50. Czaplicki CD. Contact dermatitis from Eriodictyon parryi: a novel cause of contact dermatitis in California. Wilderness Environ Med 2013;24(3):253–6.

51. Jones D. This is progress?: Surveying a Century of Native American Stories about Hair. Lion and the Unicorn 2013;37:143–56. https://doi.org/10.1353/uni.2013.0013.

52. Purnell LD, Fenkl EA. People of American Indian/Alaskan native heritage. In: Handbook for culturally competent care. Switzerland: Springer; 2019.

53. Gonzales M, King E, Bobelu J, et al. Perspectives on biological monitoring in environmental health research: a focus group study in a native american community. Int J Environ Res Public Health 2018;15(6):1129.

54. Hughes Z. More than ink: traditional tattoos roar back in Alaska. Available at: https://www.alaskapublic.org/2015/09/17/more-than-ink-traditional-tattoos-roar-back-in-alaska/. Accessed May 1, 2021.

55. Allford J. Reclaiming Inuit culture, one tattoo at a time. Available at: https://www.cnn.com/travel/article/inuit-tattoos-culture-canada/index.html. Accessed May 1, 2021.

56. Nikora LW, Rua M, Te Awekotuku N. Renewal and resistance: moko in contemporary New Zealand. J Community Appl Soc Psychol 2007;17(6):477–89.

Features of Common Skin Disorders in Pediatric Patients with Skin of Color

Uchenna K. Okoji, MPH[a], Nnenna G. Agim, MD[b], Candrice R. Heath, MD[c],*

KEYWORDS

- Skin of color • Pediatric dermatology • Ethnic skin

KEY POINTS

- Common diagnosis in pediatric dermatology may have unique clinical features in patients with skin of color
- Awareness of distinct clinical features in patients with skin of color improves outcomes for these patients
- Insight into socioeconomic factors contributing to disease incidence and treatment feasibility can inform clinical practice

INTRODUCTION

Many dermatologic conditions common in the pediatric population may have unique presentations in skin of color or occur with greater incidence. This may be due to ethnic origin, socioeconomic factors, or other influences. Awareness of the potential variations in skin of color may enhance prompt diagnosis, appropriate treatment, and/or reassurance as indicated.

NEONATAL

Transient Neonatal Pustular Melanosis

Transient neonatal pustular melanosis occurs in up to 4% of neonates and has been reported to occur more commonly in infants and toddlers with skin of color.[1] Affected children are otherwise healthy, and skin examination shows any combination of pustules, vesicles, papules, collarettes of scale, and hyperpigmented macules involving the head, lower trunk, and/or extremities. Histologically, the condition is typified by intracorneal and subcorneal neutrophilic aggregates,[2] which may also be detected by microscopic evaluation of a scraped smear. Although the eruption may persist for several months to a few years before complete resolution, unless symptomatic, treatment is not necessary. Gentle skin care may be used as supportive therapy. As with most conditions in skin of color, the associated dyspigmentation may persist long beyond the active inflammatory process.

Acropustulosis of Infancy

Acropustulosis of infancy is a chronic, recurrent, sometimes relapsing and remitting predominantly acral eruption seen in infants and toddlers. Clinical manifestations include crops of erythematous papules, frank pustules, and collarettes of scale. A diagnosis of scabies infestation may precede acropustulosis, directing the hypothesis that its origin is reactive; however, some patients do not present with this history. Its incidence is increased in populations, such as refugees and people experiencing homelessness, who are at increased risk for scabies.[3] Depending on clinical context, deficiency of interleukin-1 (IL-1) receptor antagonist, which features recurrent pustulosis, is a rare "not to miss" consideration in the differential.[4] Exclusion of bacterial, fungal, and viral infection is recommended, along with scabies preparation.

[a] Drexel University College of Medicine, 2900 West Queen Lane, Philadelphia, PA 19129, USA; [b] University of Texas Southwestern, 2350 North Stemmons Freeway, Dallas, TX 75220, USA; [c] Lewis Katz School of Medicine, Temple University, 3401 North Broad Street, 5-OPB Dermatology, Philadelphia, PA 19140, USA
* Corresponding author.
E-mail address: Nnenna.Agim@childrens.com

Dermatol Clin 40 (2022) 83–93
https://doi.org/10.1016/j.det.2021.09.002
0733-8635/22/© 2021 Elsevier Inc. All rights reserved.

Treatment, if needed, may include gentle skin care, topical corticosteroids, oral erythromycin, and oral dapsone, depending on severity.[2]

Neonatal Lupus Erythematosus

Neonatal lupus erythematosus (NLE) is a distinctive manifestation of autoantibody transfer from a mother with known or incipient connective tissue disease to her child. Maternal systemic lupus erythematosus, Sjogren syndrome, or an unspecified/overlap connective tissue disease may precede or follow the diagnosis in the neonate. Clinical features may not be present at the moment of birth, but may develop during the first year and may include periocular erythema, periocular purpura, annular or polycyclic plaques with or without prominent scale, generalized red-brown papules, focal atrophy, discoid plaques, orolabial ulceration, and reticulated erythema.[5,6] Long-term sequelae include generalized telangiectasia, atrophic scars, and postinflammatory hyperpigmentation or hypopigmentation; the dyspigmentation may be more prominent in skin of color.[7] A 2021 study of 324 patients in a single institution did not find specific associations between cardiac, hepatic, and neurologic manifestations of NLE and ethnicity in patients classified as of European (34%), non-European (48%), and mixed origin (18%).[8] Notably, the mothers in this cohort all tested positive for anti-Ro antibodies, but there was no specific description of cutaneous manifestations in alignment with ethnic origin. Anti-U1RNP antibodies have been associated with a lower risk for the conductive tissue or endomyocardial cardiac complications of NLE. Photoprotection should be encouraged along with judicious use of topical corticosteroids or calcineurin inhibitors, as spontaneous resolution is expected.[9]

INFLAMMATORY
Atopic Dermatitis

Atopic dermatitis (AD), a common chronic inflammatory disease estimated to affect up to 25% of the US population, is reported as more common in black, Asian, and Pacific Islander children.[10–12] Studies have shown that black children are 1.7 times more likely to develop AD, and Asian and Pacific Islanders are 7 times more likely to be diagnosed with AD than white children. The prevalence and persistence of the disease are highest among US urban children who are black or female.[10,13] AD is part of the "atopic triad" along with asthma and allergic rhinitis. These conditions, with similar pathophysiology, often present together in the same individual or may be elicited on review of family history.[14]

The pathogenesis of AD is complex but is thought to involve both genetic and environmental factors. Recent studies have revealed that there are differences in immune activation patterns depending on race. Although all patients with AD experience increased TH_2 activation, Asian patients with AD have more upregulation of TH_{17}/TH_{22}, and black patients have higher immunoglobulin E serum levels with no TH_{17}/TH_1 activation.[15] Clinically, this may explain variations in AD presentation, such as the psoriasiform plaques common in Asian patients.[16] These findings may have implications for AD treatment but require further investigation.[15]

AD is a heterogenous disease with a variety of clinical features and presentations. Infantile AD may present with acute/subacute eczematous dermatitis on the face or scalp, whereas childhood AD is characterized by chronic lichenified lesions on the neck, flexors, and joints.[17] Most AD lesions are pruritic with crusting and scaling.[18]

In those with skin of color, AD lesions may be follicular or papular in nature.[19] They are also more likely to experience dyschromia (hyperpigmentation or hypopigmentation) after AD.[20] In addition, AD plaques do not appear brightly erythematous, but instead feature violaceous hues. Underrecognition may lead to delayed treatment and more severe AD flares.[21] Black children are 6 times more likely than white children to have severe AD, characterized by increased surface area of disease, treatment resistance, and increased duration of flares.[18]

Treatment for AD is focused on repairing and protecting the skin's epidermal barrier, reducing pruritus, and preventing possible secondary infections. Moisturizers and emollients should be used regularly for all patients with AD. Topical corticosteroids may be applied during acute flares. Topical immunomodulators like calcineurin inhibitors (tacrolimus and pimecrolimus) or phosphodiesterase 4 inhibitor crisaborole may also be used alone or with the topical corticosteroids, based on severity.[22] For moderate to severe AD, dupilumab (IL-4 and IL-13 inhibitor) is approved down to age 6 years.[23] Phototherapy is also a treatment option, but parents and patients should be made aware that the overall skin tone may darken, as unplanned pigmentation changes may cause distress.[24]

Contact Dermatitis

Contact dermatitis is a relatively common inflammatory condition that may present as eczematous plaques in the areas of involvement. Irritant contact dermatitis can occur on initial exposure to a triggering substance and can affect most anyone regardless of race/ethnicity/heritage. This form of contact dermatitis is more likely to present acutely and with vesiculation. Allergic contact dermatitis requires repeated exposure for the type IV immunoreactivity to manifest. Atopic patients are at increased risk for contact dermatitis, the latter causing persistence of eczematous plaques or triggering atopic flares. Preemptive avoidance of potential allergens is especially important for atopic patients, as regular application of topicals means possible constant exposure to potentially allergenic compounds.

For children, the ingestion of contact allergens, such as nickel, cobalt, dyes, and fragrances, which may be part of flavoring agents, is an important consideration. Some causes of allergic and irritant contact dermatitis may be culture-specific based on unique practices. For example, preference for hair care products designed for ethnic hair variants, topical therapy for upper respiratory illness (balms containing menthol), or cleaning products for the home (eg, Pine-Sol) introduce potential allergens. Tea tree oil, lavender, balsam of Peru, and hydroperoxides of limonene are some of the allergens common to these agents.

In pediatric patients, personal care products, popular hobbies, sports equipment, outdoor activities, and the school environment are also distinct sources of specific allergens. Cocamidopropyl betaine in baby shampoo, methylisothiazolinone in diapers/wipes, liquid cleansers and slime, acetophenone azine (the 2021 allergen of the year found in shin guards and shoe foam), urushiol in poison ivy, and diffused fragrance from potent cleaning agents are some such examples. Although topical corticosteroids will improve the dermatitis, sustained resolution requires deliberate effort at identifying the causative agents and avoidance of the allergens. Patch testing allows for identification of suspected allergens and should be readily used to allow specific guidance. For patients with skin of color, postinflammatory hyperpigmentation often follows the same pattern of the originally associated dermatitis. The postinflammatory hyperpigmentation (PIHR) may be very distressing to the parents and children.

Pityriasis Rosea

Pityriasis rosea (PR) is a relatively common, self-limiting skin disease associated with the systemic reactivation of human herpesvirus-6 (HHV-6) and/or HHV-7. The inflammatory condition typically affects healthy adolescents and adults alike, ranging from ages 10 to 35 years. The incidence of PR is estimated to be 170 cases per 100,000 persons per year.[25] Although PR is more common in those with darker skin tones, it may present with a different distribution and morphology compared with those with lighter skin tones.

PR initially presents with a herald patch, a single, scaly lesion, that slowly expands. Additional lesions appear within 3 weeks of the herald patch and may persist for 4 to 10 weeks. Recent studies have found that compared with adults, children with PR have both a shorter time lapse between the presence of the herald patch and the eruption of secondary lesions (4 days compared with 2 weeks in adults) and duration of disease (on average 16 days compared with 45 days in adults).[26]

The morphologic presentation of PR on lighter skin tones and skin of color is presented in **Table 1**. The herald patch on white skin is typically erythematous with elevated scaling borders and a lighter center. In those with darker skin tones, the patch may appear brown to gray or violaceous with a central hyperpigmented necrotic area. The plaque may measure 3 cm or greater in diameter and is often the only skin manifestation for several weeks, leading to a common early misdiagnosis of tinea corporis.[27] Prodromal symptoms, such as malaise, fatigue, arthralgia, lymphadenopathy, fever, and nausea, may be present before or during the course of the skin eruptions.[28]

The distribution follows truncal cleavage lines creating a "Christmas tree" appearance regardless of ethnic skin type. Children are more likely to report pruritus.[29] Of note, black children often have more extensive distributions extending to the extremities, face, neck, and scalp with resulting postinflammatory pigmentary changes.[30]

PR bears resemblance to other hyperpigmented scaly papulosquamous eruptions, including lichen planus, guttate psoriasis, pityriasis lichenoides chronica (PLC), and secondary syphilis.[27] Lichen planus may appear more violaceous and polygonal; guttate psoriasis may follow streptococcal infection, and PLC usually has concomitant hypopigmentation and in sexually active adolescent. The presence of palmoplantar copper pennylike macules or moth-eaten alopecia suggests syphilis. In cases whereby the diagnosis is uncertain, a skin biopsy may be warranted.

As a self-limited condition, PR rarely warrants aggressive treatment; reassurance and watchful waiting are recommended. Cases with severe pruritus or extensive disease may be treated with oral antihistamines or oral corticosteroids. Acyclovir may also be a reasonable treatment option for severe cases.[31] Narrowband UV phototherapy has also been shown to be effective in reducing symptoms, but patients with skin of color should be warned about the potential for hyperpigmentation following this course of therapy.[32]

Table 1
Differences in pityriasis rosea morphology based on skin tone

	White Skin	Skin of Color
Lesion color	Salmon pink	Gray or violaceous; central necrotic-appearing hyperpigmentation
Distribution	Predominately on trunk	Trunk, extremities, face, scalp
Scale pattern	Collarette of scale on lesions	Lesions with central scale

Confluent and Reticulated Papillomatosis of Gougerot and Carteaud

Confluent and reticulated papillomatosis (CaRP) typically presents with slightly scaly, often hyperpigmented papules coalescing into reticulated plaques involving the back, chest, neck, and skin folds. Its incidence is not well described for any age group, and a loose association with type 2 diabetes mellitus in adults has been proposed. This condition tends to present around puberty and is often seen with acanthosis nigricans, which features solid plaques involving the neck and axillae. In clinical practice, the authors' observation has been that most patients are also overweight or obese and have or eventually develop insulin resistance. This important association of CaRP and glucose dysmetabolism deserves further investigation, as it may be an early cutaneous sign portending the cardiometabolic complications thereof. Treatment in adolescents is usually with a 90-day course of oral tetracyclines. These agents offer rapid improvement; however, recurrence of CaRP is common.

Discoid Lupus Erythematosus

Discoid lupus erythematosus (DLE) is a chronic autoimmune disease manifested by inflammation, which can lead to scarring and dyspigmentation. The prevalence of DLE has been described as highest in non-Latino blacks, followed by Latinos, then whites, with the lowest occurrence in those of Asian heritage.[33] Most patients with discoid lupus do not meet full criteria for systemic lupus erythematosus, but conversion is possible. This necessitates close follow-up for regular clinical and laboratory monitoring. In all patients, including those with skin of color who may not deem this usually necessary, UV protection is essential to reduce disease severity.

Tinea Versicolor

Tinea versicolor is a relatively common papulosquamous eruption occurring in children. Involvement of the neck, chest, shoulders, and back is typical, but the face may also be affected. In darker skin types, pigmentary alteration accompanies the low-level inflammation underlying this disorder. Branlike scale overlying small papules and plaques can be collected for KOH examination by microscopy; however, diagnosis is usually clinical. *Malassezia* spp play a key role in triggering the eruption and associated dyspigmentation. *Malassezia* become more abundant during puberty when androgen-dependent sebum production is enhanced; thus, this condition is most common in adolescence. Treatment is usually aimed at reducing the population of this commensal organism and any associated pruritus. Topical azoles, in cream or shampoo form, are effective and should be used for treatment and then on an intermittent basis to maintain clearance.

HAIR AND SCALP
Traction Alopecia, Traction Folliculitis, and Central Centrifugal Cicatricial Alopecia

Traction alopecia (TA) is a form of hair loss caused by repeated tension and strain imposed on hair follicles. It is most commonly seen in patients of black or African ancestry, who are more likely to wear hairstyles that tightly pull the hair shaft like braids, cornrows, and locs.[34–36] However, TA can occur in people of any race and any hair type. Children and adolescents with tightly coiled hair who wear these hairstyles have an increased risk of developing TA because their hair is more prone to breakage.[37] The use of chemicals like relaxers or dyes in the hair may also increase the risk of TA.[34]

Although TA can affect any part of the scalp, it commonly involves the hairline, hence the commonly presenting complaint of "thinning edges." The condition is biphasic in its presentation. In the early stage of TA, which is often reversible, patients may present with perifollicular erythema or follicular pustules sometimes referred to as "traction folliculitis."[36] The most critical intervention should be to discontinue use of high tension or painful hairstyles. Hair loss becomes more apparent in the later stage as indicated by the "fringe sign," retained hairs distributed along the frontotemporal portion of the scalp.[38] Once TA reaches this stage, hair loss may be permanent. Early identification and hair care habit changes during childhood may prevent TA from progressing. When approaching patients with this diagnosis, compliment first, inquire about the importance of the practices, and negotiate the move to styles with less tension, such that the patient and family feel empowered to make changes.

Central centrifugal cicatricial alopecia (CCCA) is a relatively common form of hair loss among adult black women, but importantly, may begin in later childhood. Eginli and colleagues[39,40] described biopsy-confirmed CCCA in adolescents aged 14 to 19. CCCA is characterized histopathologically by perifollicular lymphocytic inflammation and scarring of follicles on the crown of the scalp. The condition progressively expands, leading to permanent hair loss.[41]

A thorough scalp examination in those with tightly coiled hair is vital to early recognition of hair loss conditions.[42] Preceding or during the progression of CCCA, patients may also experience tenderness, scaling, and pustules at the site of hair loss.[39] Some patients with CCCA present solely with hair breakage in the crown, a form fruste of CCCA.[43] Although there is no definitive cure for CCCA, the goal of treatment is to reduce inflammation and slow down the loss of hair with the use of topical and intralesional corticosteroids, antiseborrheic shampoos, and immunomodulating oral medications.[39]

Identifying TA or CCCA early in its presentation is essential to preserving a patient's hair. All clinicians should obtain a thorough hair loss history, discuss general hair care and hairstyling practices, and provide patients with strategies to prevent further hair loss. In hair-discordant physician-patient relationships, this may require that clinicians use a culturally competent approach to examining the scalp and hair of patients with tightly coiled hair.[42]

Tinea Capitis

Tinea capitis, a fungal infection of the hair and scalp, is the most common dermatophytosis of childhood with increased prevalence among children aged 3 to 7 years.[44] The infection is caused by fungi of the Trichophyton and Microsporum genera, which are found on animals, on humans, and in soil. Current evidence suggests that children of color, particularly those of black and Hispanic heritage, are most commonly affected.[45] Other factors that predispose children to tinea capitis infection include crowded living conditions and lower socioeconomic status.[46–48]

The varied presentation of tinea capitis may present a diagnostic challenge. Depending on the degree of inflammation, tinea capitis may present clinically with (1) Diffuse scale, (2) annular plaques with scale, (3) black dots, and (4) inflammation (**Table 2**).

A focused history and physical examination are essential to making a timely accurate diagnosis. Studies have demonstrated that, among children with scalp alopecia, scale, and/or pruritus, there is a high likelihood of positive fungal culture if occipital lymphadenopathy is also present.[49]

Treating tinea capitis requires systemic, antifungal agents administered orally. Griseofulvin at a daily dose of 20 to 25 mg/kg may be required for a duration of at least 8 to 12 weeks continuously.[50] Alternatively, terbinafine, which is very efficacious against Trichophyton tonsurans, can be used in children aged 4 and older at a dose of 62.5 mg to 250 mg daily for 8 weeks, depending on body weight.[50] Antifungal shampoos may also be used to reduce the spread of fungal spores in the household; however, applications are limited to weekly or every 2 weeks to prevent dryness and attendant breakage.[50] Timely diagnosis and treatment of tinea capitis are important to prevent permanent hair loss, scarring, and spread of the infection.

FOLLICULAR
Acne: Postinflammatory Hyperpigmentation/Pomade Acne

Acne is one of the most common dermatologic conditions in both children and adults worldwide. It is a chronic disorder caused by increased sebum production, follicular hyperkeratosis, and colonization of the pilosebaceous units by Cutibacterium acnes (previously Propionibacterium acnes).[51] Reactive inflammation of these units can result in papules, pustules, comedones, nodules, or a combination.

Patients with skin of color have distinct variations in their clinical presentation of acne, for example, concentration of acneiform lesions near the hairline based on use of hair ointments, and disease sequelae (primarily dyspigmentation).[52] These patients have an increased risk of PIHR caused by the abnormal release or overproduction of melanin, usually persisting longer than active acne, often causing distress and a reduction in quality of life.[53–55] The use of moisturizing oils, emollients, and other grooming products on the scalp and face may cause the "pomade" acne subtypes described above.[56]

Treatment of acne in patients with skin of color should address both the acne and the PIHR as

Table 2
Clinical variations in tinea capitis

Clinical Presentation	Description	Common Misdiagnoses
Diffuse scale	Multiple areas of flaking, resembling generalized dandruff	Seborrheic dermatitis, atopic dermatitis
Annular plaques of scale	Well-demarcated, ring-shaped plaques	Psoriasis, seborrheic dermatitis
Black dot	Areas of hair loss with broken hair shafts; no inflammation	Alopecia areata, traction alopecia
Inflammatory	Induration or bogginess with vesicular and pustular lesions; systemic signs of infection may be present (lymphadenopathy, fever, malaise)	Posttraumatic hair conditions (eg, chemical burns), folliculitis, bacterial infection

necessary.[57] Clinicians should acknowledge that they see the pigment changes and note that the prescribed course of care will reduce inflammation and prevent PIHR exacerbations.[37] Topical retinoids are the first-line agents for treatment of acne in patients with skin of color because they may help reduce hyperpigmentation. Benzoyl peroxides and anti-inflammatory agents like dapsone and azelaic acid may also be effective, the latter especially useful because it also addresses hyperpigmentation.[52] Patients should exercise caution in the use of adjuvant therapies, such as chemical peels and laser therapy, because any resulting inflammation, peeling, or burning may cause or intensify pigment changes.[52]

Hidradenitis Suppurativa

Hidradenitis suppurativa (HS), formerly termed acne inversa, is a chronic follicular-based inflammatory disorder whose incidence increases with age. Prevalence in patients aged 10 to 14 and 15 to 17 years is estimated to increase from 27 to 114 per 100,000 persons, respectively.[58] Initial presentation occurs in the peripubertal time period as the apocrine glands are activated, and levels of tumor necrosis factor-alpha, IL-12, -17, -23, and -36a have been reported to increase. Hormonal dysregulation yielding imbalance in androgen-dependent processes likely plays a role in this age group also.[58] The axillae, buttocks, groin, intermammary, and inframammary areas are classically involved; however, severe cases may also involve the neck, flanks, and pannus.

In pediatric patients of any ethnicity, early involvement may be limited to one site, with few recurrent periodically symptomatic erythematous papules, nodules, or sinus tracts. These lesions are often mistaken for infectious folliculitis and furunculosis and treated as such, usually in an urgent care setting. About 50% of patients present with a cystic lesion that is tender half the time.[59] Short courses of oral antibiotics, incision and drainage, and topical anti-infective agents typically offer temporary relief at best, leaving families frustrated at the perceived recalcitrance. Surgical management has been estimated to have 87% complication and 7% reoperation rates.[60] Reported complications include wound dehiscence, persistent neuropathic pain, surgical site infection, granulation tissue, scar contracture, and site adhesions.[60]

Education regarding the chronic, relapsing, and remitting nature of this disease is central to any treatment plan. It is now understood that the cutaneous features of HS underlie systemic inflammatory processes, which increase risk for cardiac complications. Quality-of-life studies reveal higher morbidity among HS patients of any age compared with psoriasis, rosacea, and bullous pemphigoid[61] and 2 times the rate of depression than in unaffected adolescents.[62] Female pediatric patients seem to have a slight predominance in the Western world,[58] and obesity is a demonstrable association.[63] In a study of more than 500 pediatric patients with HS, close to 80% of whom were girls, more than half were classified as obese.[63] Polycystic ovarian and metabolic syndromes are likewise correlated, indicating that management for HS should involve global assessment of additional risk factors. Acne was found to coexist in about 33% of pediatric patients with HS, whereas hirsutism was reported in one out of 5 patients in the same cohort.[64]

Higher body mass index, anxiety, attention-deficit/hyperactivity disorder, and exposure to passive tobacco smoke were statistically more significantly associated with HS in a pediatric cohort of patients aged 5 to 17 who were greater than 90th percentile for weight at baseline.[65] Inflammatory bowel disease also occurs with greater frequency.[66] Trisomy 21 is associated with earlier onset and greater prevalence.[58,67] Early childhood intervention has the potential to stave worsening of impending cardiometabolic complications. Use of metformin in a small group pediatric patients was shown to improve outcomes.[68] The incidence of HS in patients with skin of color is estimated to occur with greater frequency compared with the other ethnicities.[63] This mirrors, to some extent, greater rates of obesity, insulin resistance, and metabolic syndrome even in the pediatric populations with skin of color.[69] Obesity rates were calculated as between 2- and 3-fold higher in pediatric HS patients in one study.[70] Although there are some genetic underpinnings possibly explaining occurrence in families (<10%), the contribution of modifiable environmental factors cannot be dismissed. Affected patients and their families should be counseled regarding a low-carbohydrate diet, referred to nutritionists, and encouraged to engage in regular physical activity.

PIGMENTARY DISORDERS
Vitiligo

Vitiligo is an autoimmune condition in which melanocytes are rendered ineffective under cytotoxic T-cell attack. The ensuing loss of melanin production causes pigment dilution as first evidenced by hypopigmentation, evolving into complete depigmentation. Trichrome vitiligo demonstrates this process. The patient's intrinsic background pigmentation does not usually make clinical detection challenging in darker skin types, given the ready contrast between pigmented and depigmented areas. Wood's lamp is more important for delineating mucosal involvement, confetti lesions indicating incipient extension, and signs of recovery (diminution of depigmentation, follicular repigmentation). This ease of diagnosis belies the significant social and psychological consequences of the contrast between affected and unaffected skin readily on display to the patient and public.

For children able to use the technology, phototherapy is an option for treatment, although insurance coverage varies. Treatment options continue to evolve with investigation of the JAK/STAT pathways. Total depigmentation is a viable option rarely used in children. This option however should be carefully considered given the social and psychological consequences during evolution of identity during these vulnerable years. There is no set protocol for pediatric depigmentation; thus, such a decision should be reserved for patients with 50% to 60% or more body surface area of pigment loss and education and discussion with the family.

Postinflammatory Hyperpigmentation and Hypopigmentation

Postinflammatory hyperpigmentation
(PIHR is a reactive response of the skin resulting in hypermelanosis following cutaneous trauma or injury. It is a common sequalae of inflammatory skin conditions like acne, folliculitis, and AD in pediatric and adults patients with skin of color.[57,71] PIHR is one of the most common dermatologic complaints in patients with skin of color.[72]

The pathogenesis of PIHR is thought to consist of 2 different processes at the epidermal and dermal layer. Epidermal hypermelanosis is caused by the overstimulation of melanocytes by leukotrienes, prostaglandins, and cytokines after an inflammatory response.[73-75] Dermal hypermelanosis involves the destruction of melanin-containing keratinocytes at the basal layer and the phagocytosis of this melanin by macrophages in the upper dermis.[76,77] PIHR presents as deeply pigmented macules or patches on the skin that patients often find distressing. Left untreated, these pigmentary changes may take months to years to fade away.[72]

Treatment plans for PIHR should first address the underlying inflammatory condition and promote strategies to prevent further pigmentary changes. Clinicians should follow guidelines for treating the inflammatory skin condition and use a patient-centered approach for treatment options. Patients should be advised on gentle skin care routines that involve gentle cleansers and moisturizers to minimize further irritation or dryness that may exacerbate PIHR.[57]

Photoprotection, either sunscreen or barriers, such as clothing, hats, and sunglasses, may also prevent further darkening and reduce the duration of PIHR. When selecting sunscreen for patients with skin of color, avoid recommending products that leave an opaque white residue on the skin.[57] Once the underlying condition has been appropriately managed, topical agents can be used to lighten areas of the skin with PIHR (see later discussion). Adolescents with concurrent PIHR and acne can incorporate alpha-hydroxy acid–based cleansers, expert applied glycolic and salicylic acid chemical peels, and cosmeceuticals to treat PIHR.[57] Cosmeceuticals include over-the-counter or prescription products containing kojic acid, niacinamide, arbutin, licorice, and/or a variety of other agents. Topical ammonium lactate 12% can be used to replenish skin moisture and decrease corneocyte adhesion in nonfacial areas, potentially dissipating pigment appearance or enhancing penetration of other skin-lightening agents.[78]

The gold standard for skin lightening is topical hydroquinone; however, it is not approved for use in children.[71,79] Parents of children with PIHR may elect to use hydroquinone on their children if other therapies (photoprotection, gentle skin care, and time) are not successful, but they should be counseled on the potential risks of ochronosis, and off-label use should be emphasized.[57] Alternative therapies, such as mequinol, azelaic acid, kojic acid, retinoids, and procedures like chemexfoliation and laser therapy, have been used in adults with varied success, but have not yet been approved for children. Although these therapies have been shown to improve PIHR, no ideal combination has been determined.[80] Patients should be cautioned about potential adverse effects of these therapies that may lead to further irritation, inflammation, and sometimes worsening of PIHR.[72]

Post-inflammatory hypopigmentation

Like PIHR, postinflammatory hypopigmentation (PIHO) is also an acquired condition as a result of cutaneous injury. It occurs in all skin types but is more common and visible on patients with darker skin tones.[81] PIHO can be caused by inflammatory skin disorders, such as AD, pityriasis alba, seborrheic dermatitis, as well as neoplastic conditions like hypopigmented mycosis fungoides, which has a higher incidence in patients with skin of color.[81,82]

Although the pathogenesis of PIHO is still unclear, leading theories point to processes that reduce the expression and presentation of melanin either by reduced melanin production and distribution or by melanocyte destruction.[83] The clinical presentation of PIHO varies in the size, distribution, and extent of hypopigmented lesions (ranging from hypopigmentation to complete depigmentation). These lesions may sometimes exist alongside those from the underlying inflammatory disorder. In patients with recently tanned skin from sun exposure, PIHO may appear to be more severe than it is in actuality, so it is important to inquire about the patient's "normal" skin tone or search for it by examining non–sun-exposed areas like the proximal medial arm.

Wood's lamp examination can be used to differentiate hypopigmentation from depigmentation as well as distinguish PIHO from other disorders that present similarly and are frequently seen in pediatric patients with skin of color. For example, under Wood's lamp, progressive macular hypomelanosis has a red fluorescence, whereas pityriasis versicolor is orange.[84] In cases whereby a diagnosis is unclear and there is clinical suspicion for a more worrisome condition, such as mycosis fungoides or leprosy, a skin biopsy can be obtained.

Treatment of PIHO requires addressing the underlying cause of the cutaneous injury. In some cases, this can lead to resolution of the pigmentary changes within weeks or months. If PIHO persists, additional interventions for the underlying conditions can be used.[81] For example, the hypopigmentation associated with tinea versicolor or infantile seborrheic dermatitis responds well to natural sunlight, whereas that associated with PLC or hypopigmented mycosis fungoides requires narrow-band-UV-B. For most inflammatory conditions, over time, with control of the underlying diagnosis, normal pigmentation returns. Thus, clinicians should counsel patients on striking a balance between pigment restoration and inducing hyperpigmentation when developing a treatment plan.

SUMMARY

Pediatric patients represent an important and unique subset of the population of skin of color. Although similar conditions present across all spectrums of skin color in childhood and adolescence, varying morphologies exist based on background skin tone; such variance may delay diagnosis. Melanocyte biology, socioeconomic factors, such as urban residence, and cultural practices, for example, based on hair texture, may be linked directly to such presentations. Highlighting these features in children with skin of color, where present, will, it is hoped, improve awareness, improve diagnosis, and prevent treatment delay.

CLINICS CARE POINTS

- Atopic dermatitis may present with follicular prominence or papular morphology in pediatric patients with skin of color. Erythema appears violaceous.

- When there is increased suspicion for contact allergy, refer for or perform patch testing.

- Traction alopecia is a biphasic alopecia. Initially, it is reversible with early intervention and permanently scarring in later stages. Hairstyle modification during childhood can prevent devastating future permanent hair loss.

DISCLOSURE

The authors have nothing to disclose.

REFERENCES

1. Chadha A, Jahnke M. Common neonatal rashes. Pediatr Ann 2019;48(1):e16–22.
2. Chia PS, Leung C, Hsu YL, et al. An infant with transient neonatal pustular melanosis presenting as pustules. Pediatr Neonatol 2010;51(6):356–8.
3. Good LM, Good TJ, High WA. Infantile acropustulosis in internationally adopted children. J Am Acad Dermatol 2011;65(4):763–71.
4. Minkis K, Aksentijevich I, Goldbach-Mansky R, et al. Interleukin 1 receptor antagonist deficiency presenting as infantile pustulosis mimicking infantile pustular psoriasis. Arch Dermatol 2012;148(6):747–52.
5. Paller A, Mancini A. Collagen vascular disorders. In: Hurwitz clinical pediatric dermatology. 5th edition. Elvsevier; 2016. p. 640.
6. Drohan A, Snyder A, Plante J, et al. Neonatal lupus erythematosus presenting as orolabial ulcerations: two cases and a review of the literature. Pediatr Dermatol 2021. https://doi.org/10.1111/pde.14555.
7. Wei-Yi Wee L, Liew WK, Jean-Aan Koh M. Purpuric lesions and atrophic scars in a neonate. JAAD Case Rep 2021;9:48–51.
8. Diaz T, Dominguez D, Jaeggi E, et al. Ethnicity and neonatal lupus erythematosus manifestations risk in a large multi-ethnic cohort. J Rheumatol 2021. https://doi.org/10.3899/jrheum.201338.
9. Wu J, Berk-Krauss J, Glick SA. Neonatal lupus erythematosus. JAMA Dermatol 2021. https://doi.org/10.1001/jamadermatol.2021.0041.
10. Kaufman BP, Guttman-Yassky E, Alexis AF. Atopic dermatitis in diverse racial and ethnic groups-variations in epidemiology, genetics, clinical presentation and treatment. Exp Dermatol 2018;27(4):340–57.
11. Eichenfield LF, Tom WL, Chamlin SL, et al. Guidelines of care for the management of atopic dermatitis: section 1. Diagnosis and assessment of atopic dermatitis. J Am Acad Dermatol 2014;70(2):338–51.
12. Hanifin JM, Cooper KD, Ho VC, et al. Guidelines of care for atopic dermatitis, developed in accordance with the American Academy of Dermatology (AAD)/American Academy of Dermatology Association "Administrative Regulations for Evidence-Based Clinical Practice Guidelines. J Am Acad Dermatol 2004;50(3):391–404.
13. McKenzie C, Silverberg JI. The prevalence and persistence of atopic dermatitis in urban United States children. Ann Allergy Asthma Immunol 2019;123(2):173–8.e1.
14. Stone KD. Atopic diseases of childhood. Curr Opin Pediatr 2002;14(5):634–46.
15. Brunner PM, Guttman-Yassky E. Racial differences in atopic dermatitis. Ann Allergy Asthma Immunol 2019;122(5):449–55.
16. Chan TC, Sanyal RD, Pavel AB, et al. Atopic dermatitis in Chinese patients shows T(H)2/T(H)17 skewing with psoriasiform features. J Allergy Clin Immunol 2018;142(3):1013–7.
17. Browning J. Dermatology edited by Jean L. Bolognia Julie V. Schaffer Lorenzo Cerroni Fourth edition China: Elsevier, 2018. Pediatr Dermatol 2018;35(2):289.
18. Poladian K, De Souza B, McMichael AJ. Atopic dermatitis in adolescents with skin of color. Cutis 2019;104(3):164–8.
19. Julián-Gónzalez RE, Orozco-Covarrubias L, Durán-McKinster C, et al. Less common clinical manifestations of atopic dermatitis: prevalence by age. Pediatr Dermatol 2012;29(5):580–3.
20. Maymone MBC, Watchmaker JD, Dubiel M, et al. Common skin disorders in pediatric skin of color. J Pediatr Health Care 2019;33(6):727–37.
21. Ben-Gashir MA, Hay RJ. Reliance on erythema scores may mask severe atopic dermatitis in black children compared with their white counterparts. Br J Dermatol 2002;147(5):920–5.
22. Paller AS, Tom WL, Lebwohl MG, et al. Efficacy and safety of crisaborole ointment, a novel, nonsteroidal phosphodiesterase 4 (PDE4) inhibitor for the topical treatment of atopic dermatitis (AD) in children and adults. J Am Acad Dermatol 2016;75(3):494–503.e6.
23. Guttman-Yassky E, Bissonnette R, Ungar B, et al. Dupilumab progressively improves systemic and cutaneous abnormalities in patients with atopic dermatitis. J Allergy Clin Immunol 2019;143(1):155–72.
24. Sidbury R, Davis DM, Cohen DE, et al. Guidelines of care for the management of atopic dermatitis: section 3. Management and treatment with phototherapy and systemic agents. J Am Acad Dermatol 2014;71(2):327–49.
25. Chuh AA, Dofitas BL, Comisel GG, et al. Interventions for pityriasis rosea. Cochrane Database Syst Rev 2007;(2):Cd005068.
26. Drago F, Ciccarese G, Broccolo F, et al. Pityriasis rosea in children: clinical features and laboratory investigations. Dermatology 2015;231(1):9–14.
27. Drago F, Ciccarese G, Rebora A, et al. Pityriasis rosea: a comprehensive classification. Dermatology 2016;232(4):431–7.
28. Rebora A, Drago F, Broccolo F. Pityriasis rosea and herpesviruses: facts and controversies. Clin Dermatol 2010;28(5):497–501.
29. Gündüz O, Ersoy-Evans S, Karaduman A. Childhood pityriasis rosea. Pediatr Dermatol 2009;26(6):750–1.

30. Amer A, Fischer H, Li X. The natural history of pityriasis rosea in black American children: how correct is the "classic" description? Arch Pediatr Adolesc Med 2007;161(5):503–6.

31. Villalon-Gomez JM. Pityriasis rosea: diagnosis and treatment. Am Fam Physician 2018;97(1):38–44.

32. Jairath V, Mohan M, Jindal N, et al. Narrowband UVB phototherapy in pityriasis rosea. Indian Dermatol Online J 2015;6(5):326–9.

33. Izmirly P, Buyon J, Belmont HM, et al. Population-based prevalence and incidence estimates of primary discoid lupus erythematosus from the Manhattan Lupus Surveillance Program. Lupus Sci Med 2019;6(1):e000344. Erratum in: Lupus Sci Med. 2019 Nov 14;6(1):e000344corr1. PMID: 31798917; PMCID: PMC6827754.

34. Khumalo NP, Jessop S, Gumedze F, et al. Hairdressing and the prevalence of scalp disease in African adults. Br J Dermatol 2007;157(5):981–8.

35. Khumalo NP, Jessop S, Gumedze F, et al. Hairdressing is associated with scalp disease in African schoolchildren. Br J Dermatol 2007;157(1):106–10.

36. Lawson CN, Hollinger J, Sethi S, et al. Updates in the understanding and treatments of skin & hair disorders in women of color. Int J Womens Dermatol 2017;3(1 Suppl):S21–37.

37. Grayson C, Heath C. Tips for addressing common conditions affecting pediatric and adolescent patients with skin of color. Pediatr Dermatol 2021. https://doi.org/10.1111/pde.14525.

38. Samrao A, Price VH, Zedek D, et al. The "fringe sign" - a useful clinical finding in traction alopecia of the marginal hair line. Dermatol Online J 2011;17(11):1.

39. Aguh C, McMichael A. Central centrifugal cicatricial alopecia. JAMA Dermatol 2020;156(9):1036.

40. Eginli AN, Dlova NC, McMichael A. Central centrifugal cicatricial alopecia in children: a case series and review of the literature. Pediatr Dermatol 2017;34(2):133–7.

41. Dlova NC, Salkey KS, Callender VD, et al. Central centrifugal cicatricial alopecia: new insights and a call for action. J Investig Dermatol Symp Proc 2017;18(2):S54–6.

42. Grayson C, Heath C. An approach to examining tightly coiled hair among patients with hair loss in race-discordant patient-physician interactions. JAMA Dermatol 2021. https://doi.org/10.1001/jamadermatol.2021.0338.

43. Callender VD, Wright DR, Davis EC, et al. Hair breakage as a presenting sign of early or occult central centrifugal cicatricial alopecia: clinicopathologic findings in 9 patients. Arch Dermatol 2012;148(9):1047–52.

44. Michaels BD, Del Rosso JQ. Tinea capitis in infants: recognition, evaluation, and management suggestions. J Clin Aesthet Dermatol 2012;5(2):49–59.

45. Alvarez M, Silverberg N. Tinea capitis. In: Dermatology for skin of color, vol 1, 2 edition. McGraw Hill Medical; 2009. p. 800.

46. Ajello L. Geographic distribution and prevalence of the dermatophytes. Ann N Y Acad Sci 1960;89:30–8.

47. Fuller LC, Child FC, Midgley G, et al. Scalp ringworm in south-east London and an analysis of a cohort of patients from a paediatric dermatology department. Br J Dermatol 2003;148(5):985–8.

48. Honig PJ. Tinea capitis: recommendations for school attendance. Pediatr Infect Dis J 1999;18(2):211–4.

49. Hubbard TW. The predictive value of symptoms in diagnosing childhood tinea capitis. Arch Pediatr Adolesc Med 1999;153(11):1150–3.

50. Möhrenschlager M, Seidl HP, Ring J, et al. Pediatric tinea capitis: recognition and management. Am J Clin Dermatol 2005;6(4):203–13.

51. Williams HC, Dellavalle RP, Garner S. Acne vulgaris. Lancet 2012;379(9813):361–72.

52. Alexis AF. Acne vulgaris in skin of color: understanding nuances and optimizing treatment outcomes. J Drugs Dermatol 2014;13(6):s61–5.

53. Perkins AC, Cheng CE, Hillebrand GG, et al. Comparison of the epidemiology of acne vulgaris among Caucasian, Asian, Continental Indian and African American women. J Eur Acad Dermatol Venereol 2011;25(9):1054–60.

54. Alexis AF, Harper JC, Stein Gold LF, et al. Treating acne in patients with skin of color. Semin Cutan Med Surg 2018;37(3s):S71–3.

55. Darji K, Varade R, West D, et al. Psychosocial impact of postinflammatory hyperpigmentation in patients with acne vulgaris. J Clin Aesthet Dermatol 2017;10(5):18–23.

56. Davis EC, Callender VD. A review of acne in ethnic skin: pathogenesis, clinical manifestations, and management strategies. J Clin Aesthet Dermatol 2010;3(4):24–38.

57. Heath CR. Managing postinflammatory hyperpigmentation in pediatric patients with skin of color. Cutis 2019;103(2):71–3.

58. Choi E, Ting OX, Chandran NS. Hidradenitis suppurativa in pediatric patients. J Am Acad Dermatol 2020. https://doi.org/10.1016/j.jaad.2020.08.045.

59. Liy-Wong C, Kim M, Kirkorian AY, et al. Hidradenitis suppurativa in the pediatric population: an international, multicenter, retrospective, cross-sectional study of 481 pediatric patients. JAMA Dermatol 2021;157(4):385–91.

60. Ge S, Ngaage LM, Orbay H, et al. Surgical management of pediatric hidradenitis suppurativa: a case series and review of the literature. Ann Plast Surg 2020;84(5):570–4.

61. Alavi A, Anooshirvani N, Kim WB, et al. Quality-of-life impairment in patients with hidradenitis suppurativa: a Canadian study. Am J Clin Dermatol 2015;16(1):61–5.

62. McAndrew R, Lopes F, Sebastian K, et al. Quality of life in hidradenitis suppurativa: a cross-sectional study of a pediatric population. J Am Acad Dermatol 2021;84(3):829–30.

63. Reichert B, Fernandez Faith E, Harfmann K. Weight counseling in pediatric hidradenitis suppurativa patients. Pediatr Dermatol 2020;37(3):480–3.

64. Riis PT, Saunte DM, Sigsgaard V, et al. Clinical characteristics of pediatric hidradenitis suppurativa: a cross-sectional multicenter study of 140 patients. Arch Dermatol Res 2020;312(10):715–24.

65. Lindsø Andersen P, Kromann C, Fonvig CE, et al. Hidradenitis suppurativa in a cohort of overweight and obese children and adolescents. Int J Dermatol 2019. https://doi.org/10.1111/ijd.14639.

66. Lloyd-McLennan AM, Ali S, Kittler NW. Prevalence of inflammatory bowel disease among pediatric patients with hidradenitis suppurativa and the potential role of screening with fecal calprotectin. Pediatr Dermatol 2021;38(1):98–102.

67. Sechi A, Guglielmo A, Patrizi A, et al. Disseminate recurrent folliculitis and hidradenitis suppurativa are associated conditions: results from a retrospective study of 131 patients with down syndrome and a cohort of 12,351 pediatric controls. Dermatol Pract Concept 2019;9(3):187–94.

68. Moussa C, Wadowski L, Price H, et al. Metformin as adjunctive therapy for pediatric patients with hidradenitis suppurativa. J Drugs Dermatol 2020;19(12):1231–4.

69. Rodríguez-Zuñiga MJM, García-Perdomo HA, Ortega-Loayza AG. Association between hidradenitis suppurativa and metabolic syndrome: a systematic review and meta-analysis. Actas Dermosifiliogr 2019;110(4):279–88. Asociación entre la hidradenitis supurativa y el síndrome metabólico: Revisión sistemática y metaanálisis.

70. Balgobind A, Finelt N, Strunk A, et al. Association between obesity and hidradenitis suppurativa among children and adolescents: a population-based analysis in the United States. J Am Acad Dermatol 2020;82(2):502–4.

71. Davis EC, Callender VD. Postinflammatory hyperpigmentation: a review of the epidemiology, clinical features, and treatment options in skin of color. J Clin Aesthet Dermatol 2010;3(7):20–31.

72. Callender VD, St Surin-Lord S, Davis EC, et al. Postinflammatory hyperpigmentation: etiologic and therapeutic considerations. Am J Clin Dermatol 2011;12(2):87–99.

73. Tomita Y, Maeda K, Tagami H. Melanocyte-stimulating properties of arachidonic acid metabolites: possible role in postinflammatory pigmentation. Pigment Cell Res 1992;5(5 Pt 2):357–61.

74. Ortonne JP. Retinoic acid and pigment cells: a review of in-vitro and in-vivo studies. Br J Dermatol 1992;127(Suppl 41):43–7.

75. Taylor S, Grimes P, Lim J, et al. Postinflammatory hyperpigmentation. J Cutan Med Surg 2009;13(4):183–91.

76. Nordlund JJ, Abdel-Malek ZA. Mechanisms for postinflammatory hyperpigmentation and hypopigmentation. Prog Clin Biol Res 1988;256:219–36.

77. Masu S, Seiji M. Pigmentary incontinence in fixed drug eruptions. Histologic and electron microscopic findings. J Am Acad Dermatol 1983;8(4):525–32.

78. Heath, Candrice "Managing Post-inflammatory Hyperpigmentation in Pediatric Patients With Skin of Color" Cutis. Perrigo New York, Inc. 2019 February;103(2):71-73

79. Grimes PE. Management of hyperpigmentation in darker racial ethnic groups. Semin Cutan Med Surg 2009;28(2):77–85.

80. Shokeen D. Postinflammatory hyperpigmentation in patients with skin of color. Cutis 2016;97(1):E9–11.

81. Madu PN, Syder N, Elbuluk N. Postinflammatory hypopigmentation: a comprehensive review of treatments. J Dermatolog Treat 2020;20:1–5.

82. Hinds GA, Heald P. Cutaneous T-cell lymphoma in skin of color. J Am Acad Dermatol 2009;60(3):359–75 [quiz 376–8].

83. Carlson JA, Grabowski R, Mu XC, et al. Possible mechanisms of hypopigmentation in lichen sclerosus. Am J Dermatopathol 2002;24(2):97–107.

84. Vachiramon V, Thadanipon K. Postinflammatory hypopigmentation. Clin Exp Dermatol 2011;36(7):708–14.

Tips, Tricks, and Pearls to Expertly Treat Common Pediatric Dermatologic Conditions

James Treat, MD

KEYWORDS

- Pediatrics • Dermatology • Atopic dermatitis • Hemangiomas • Psoriasis • Molluscum
- Skin of color

KEY POINTS

- Allergic conotact dermatitis is under-recognized in children with atopic dermatitis. Clinicians should try to limit the exposure of chidren to fragrancess and preservatives.
- There are many systemic medicaitons now available for psoriasis and when children have ssignificant psoriasis and are not adequately treated by topical or light therapy, systemic therapy shoould be considered.
- Clinical clue to hemangiomas including that they are not fully formed at birth, may have a ring of pallor around them and go through a typical growth pattern help to establish the diagnosis and guide therapy.

I would like to start this chapter by acknowledging that the field of pediatric dermatology is filled with truly outstanding clinicians, communicators, and educators. I have learned from so many great mentors who recognize subtle clinical differences and have mastered how to communicate with families. I am honored to write a chapter based on the tips and tricks that I have picked up from these amazing teachers and from the patients and families for whom I have had the privilege to care.

I have divided this chapter based on a handful of common pediatric dermatologic diseases and what I see as some of the main clinical and therapeutic tips and tricks that have helped me in my practice.

ATOPIC DERMATITIS

Atopic dermatitis (AD) is very common in children. Most AD is mild and can be treated with topical steroids and moisturizers. AD is at its core a barrier problem with an exaggerated immune response.

Moisturizing to help heal the skin barrier and topical immunomodulatory agents such as steroids and calcineurin inhibitors to decrease excessive secretion of TH2 cytokines in response to skin irritation are key to therapy.[1] It is also imperative to have a maintenance plan. Options for maintenance include the following:

- Applying the topical steroid that was used for the flare 2 times weekly in areas most likely to flare.[2]
- Use of a calcineurin inhibitor or crisaborole to prevent flares is helpful when there are focal areas that tend to flare (especially if these flares are on sensitive sites such as the face, folds, or anogenital area) where consistent use of topical steroids has more risk of thinned skin.
- Mixing a low potency topical steroid with a moisturizer used every other day is best for prevention of widespread AD.

University of Pennsylvania, Philadelphia, PA, USA
E-mail address: treat@email.chop.edu

Dermatol Clin 40 (2022) 95–102
https://doi.org/10.1016/j.det.2021.09.009
0733-8635/22/© 2021 Elsevier Inc. All rights reserved.

derm.theclinics.com

When AD is severe and recalcitrant to appropriate strength topical steroids along with aggressive moisturizing and gentle skin care, factors that may be exacerbating the disease should be sought. Allergic contact dermatitis is underrecognized in AD.[3] If children have widespread disease consider allergens that may be used all over the body, such as sorbitan sesquioleate and propylene glycol that may be in the topical medicines. Lanolin or methylisothiazolinone may be in moisturizers or soaps. Fragrances can be in almost any product. Allergens such as fragrances that are on caretakers may be transferred onto children and should be eliminated. Another possible source of recalcitrant AD is infection. Children with AD can easily become infected with *Staphylococcus aureus* or *Streptococcus pyogenes* and can be recurrently infected with herpes simplex.[4] Attempting to prevent the infections with dilute bleach baths that may decrease colonization and prophylactic acyclovir can help prevent flares of AD associated with herpes reactivation.[5] Other possible causes of flares include itching associated with environmental allergies, immunodeficiencies, and rarely food allergies.

When good skin care, appropriate topical steroids, and avoidance of triggers are not helpful enough, systemic therapy should be offered. The decision to initiate systemic therapy for AD should be based on the severity of disease but also the impact on the child's life. AD can be really impactful on children and families. The constant itching and challenges posed by complicated skin regimens combined with lack of sleep for the children and their parents can be devastating. Children often wake up in the night and come to their parent's room and co-sleep, which also has a broad negative impact.[6] There is much more recognition of the associated behavioral health and school issues caused by AD. These include anxiety, depression, and poor school performance.

Phototherapy and systemic therapy such as dupilumab (on label for those aged 6 years and older) or methotrexate or cyclosporine (both off label) can be life changing for children who are severely affected both physically and emotionally by their AD. If effective, children often become less socially withdrawn and thrive more in relationships and academics. These are important points to relay to parents who are often afraid of using systemic medications. Usually the risk of not using a systemic drug and having children continue in their state of extreme itchiness and behavioral dysphoria is significantly higher than the risk of the medications.

JUVENILE PLANTAR DERMATOSIS

Juvenile plantar dermatosis (JPD) is really impactful on children and tends to be misdiagnosed and incorrectly treated because it is not just AD on the plantar feet. The scaling of JPD is unique in that it looks similar to parchment paper that then fissures and bleeds. Typically, it is worst at the base of the great toe, ball of the foot, and sometimes heel. Many clinicians assume this is tinea but the lack of involvement in between the toes and typical parchment paper appearance helps differentiate it. If unsure, a potassium hydroxide (KOH) prep confirms the absence of dermatophytes. JPD is not as much of an inflammatory condition as an adverse response to repeated wetting and drying.[7] Therefore, topical steroids are not very helpful. Parents want to know the quick fix prescription they can use to cure it but the most effective intervention is consistent prevention of wetting and drying including controlling sweating. Keeping the skin moisturized but not sweaty or wet is the key. If summer/sandal type shoes are worn, ideally socks should be worn also (not always stylish but very helpful). Although the feet may still sweat and the socks may need to be changed, the cotton can absorb the sweat and pull away from the skin at least temporarily. If the wetness is from sweating, then topical antiperspirants can help. But, caution, if applying aluminum chloride or similar antiperspirant to the feet when actively fissured, it will burn, so ideally antiperspirants are used preventatively. Some children prefer to just be bare foot, and this is very reasonable as long as the skin is also moisturized.

PSORIASIS

Similar to AD, psoriasis can also have a serious negative effect on children's lives. Therefore, many of the same arguments about the utility and benefits of systemic medications outlined earlier for AD apply also to psoriasis. There are a few psoriasis tips and tricks that are specific to children. Infants often present with psoriasis in their perineum thought to be due to koebnerization from diapers. Children get more facial psoriasis than adults.[8] Discrete scaling plaques on the upper eyelid is often one of the first manifestations of psoriasis in children, possibly due to koebnerization from eye rubbing. Children and parents may not know to divulge the itching and scaling rashes that occur on the penis, labia, and intergluteal cleft unless asked directly. Children also have a more direct link between *Group A Streptococcal* infection and flares of psoriasis than adults.[9]

Recurrent guttate psoriasis in children should prompt a clinical evaluation for strep. Older children and adolescents often get pharyngeal strep, whereas younger children may be infected in the anogenital area including the anus, vulva, and penis. Therefore, examination and culture of both areas is key in younger children especially.

In terms of systemic therapy, therapeutic benefit of a particular medication needs to be balanced with the frequency of blood draws and injections. A few pearls on using systemic medications:

- Cyclosporine and acitretin tend to work quickly in patients with pustular psoriasis[10]
- Acitretin is restricted in women of child-bearing potential due to risk of fetus potentially for years after use but also make sure mothers of children are not handling the medicine due to risk to a fetus if they absorbed it.
- Note for methotrexate, if bloodwork is done within a few days of the dose, the liver functions may be elevated and spur dosing changes that are unnecessary.
- Subcutaneous methotrexate is a reasonable option to assure absorption and if there is significant nausea with the oral version.
- Etanercept is approved for use by the Food and Drug Administration (FDA) for psoriasis for children 4 years of age and older. The recommendation for the varicella and measles/mumps/rubella vaccinations (both are live attenuated and not recommended to be given to children on immunosuppressing medications). So ideally these vaccination boosters are given before starting a biological medication.
- Ixekizumab, ustekinumab, and secukinumab have fortunately become approved by the FDA for children 6 years and older.
- Ustekinumab is given only every 3 months (after loading dose), which can help with needle phobia.

MOLLUSCUM CONTAGIOSUM

Molluscum is frustrating to both parents and practitioners. Diagnostically, molluscum is usually not a challenge, especially when the presentation is classic as flesh-colored umbilicated papules. It is less well recognized that molluscum can also present as cysts, inflamed papules, pustules, and abscesses. When in doubt, a few techniques can help confirm the diagnosis:

- Dermoscopy of molluscum usually shows white/yellow lobules.[11] Tip: use noncontact dermoscopy or use a throw-away shield to prevent spread to other patients.
- KOH: if there is any extrusion from a cyst or pustular lesion, a KOH prep can reveal Henderson Patterson bodies (**Fig. 1**).
- Side-lighting molluscum usually reveals a slight indentation or a centrally extruding white core. When using liquid nitrogen, the central dell of the molluscum is highlighted (**Fig. 2**).
- Scan for scarring: resolved lesions may leave around 1 to 2 mm indentations that indicate that molluscum were there, suggesting the diagnosis when only non-classic inflamed or pustular lesions are present.

Molluscum can also lead to multiple other dermatologic conditions that are helpful to recognize. The immune response to molluscum can lead to a hypersensitivity or inflammatory reaction around molluscum. One of the more common presentations is a seemingly out of place, spontaneous area of dermatitis in an isolated antecubital fossa or an isolated axillary vault or inguinal fold; this often occurs in patients who may have a remote history or no history of AD.[12] The dermatitis is often itchy and only on very close inspection tiny molluscum can be found in the center. The clinical differential of an isolated patch of dermatitis includes, among other things, allergic contact dermatitis, irritant contact dermatitis, AD, and, as described, molluscum dermatitis. In addition, there can be a much broader hypersensitivity reaction of fine papules over the elbows, knees, and cheeks; this is likely an id reaction that spares the trunk in a classic Gianotti-Crosti pattern, which is underrecognized in the setting of molluscum

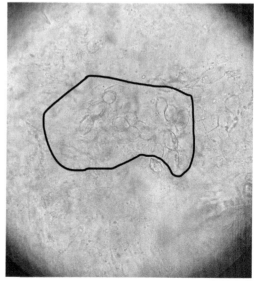

Fig. 1. Henderson-Patterson bodies.

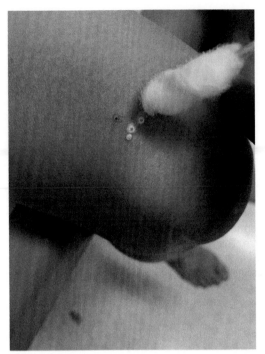

Fig. 2. Freezing mollusscum lightly highlightss umbilication.

contagiosum.[13] The lesions of Gianotti-Crosti are small papules that are dome-shaped and mimic the molluscum and is especially disconcerting to parents. Gianotti-Crosti syndrome occurs usually at the end of the course of the molluscum, and the parents often misperceive the papules as rapidly spreading molluscum when in fact it is usually the beginning of the end.

When treating molluscum it is vital to do what is in the best interest of the child and not to treat too aggressively to appease the parent especially because this is self-resolving in most. For instance, curettage or liquid nitrogen for multiple lesions can be painful and traumatizing especially in younger children who cannot assent to the procedure. Cantharidin is often the happy medium of an effective therapeutic that is not painful. Caution when applying this—less is much, much more—limit application to the top of the molluscum, avoiding surrounding normal skin. I typically do not treat lesions that are underneath underwear because therapy in occluded areas can lead to excessive blistering and pain. One of the other main options for therapy is to simply treat the dermatitis or secondary changes that happen around the molluscum. The itch is often what is most distressing to the child. It is also important to understand that once the inflammatory reaction to the molluscum is exuberant, usually the

infection will be gone within 1 to 2 months so watchful waiting is appropriate. Tretinoin is often effective for facial lesions but should be used only directly on top of the molluscum with application by a toothpick or cotton swab to avoid irritating neighboring skin.[14] Imiquimod has been proved ineffective for molluscum in a large trial, and this study is referenced in the package insert.

Verruca Vulgaris

Warts are a nuisance to the patient, their parents, and often the provider because they are recalcitrant to therapy, ubiquitous, and socially stigmatizing. For individual or a few warts, liquid nitrogen is still usually the therapy for choice unless children are too young or too anxious; then, local therapy with topical salicylic acid and tape is often effective. For multiple warts especially in challenging to treat areas, injecting candida antigen into a few warts can help bolster the immune response against all of them.[15] Although kids may hate the idea of an injection, the actual pain from the injection is often less than that from cryotherapy. Warts can be recalcitrant to many therapies especially in patients with immune deficiency. Off label options include topical cidofovir between 1% and 3% or a proprietary mixture of topical 5-Fluorouracil and salicylic acid that must be compounded.[16,17] Caution is advised, as the ingestion of any of these compounded agents may be dangerous and use should be avoided around pregnant people or for young children who may ingest them.

HEMANGIOMAS

There are a few helpful tips and tricks for both diagnosing and treating hemangiomas. First, it is important to recognize that infantile hemangiomas go through a very typical growth pattern of absence (or unapparent) at birth or at the most presenting as a telangiectatic or bruised red patch with vasoconstriction. If there is any substance or they are fully formed at birth then the diagnosis is likely to be another type of vascular or malignant tumor. There are some variants of hemangiomas including abortive hemangiomas or infantile hemangiomas with minimal or arrested growth (IHMAG), which are telangiectatic patches often present at birth with a rim of vasoconstriction.[18] In the first weeks and months small papules of hemangioma tend to grow within the lesion and offer a clue to confirm the diagnosis. It is of paramount importance to recognize these types of hemangiomas because they can be associated with hemangioma syndromes (Posterior fossa malformations, Hemangiomas of the face [or neck], Arterial anomalies, Cardiac anomalies, and Eye abnormalities [PHACE] syndrome and Lower body hemangioma, Urogenital abnormalities, Myelopathy, Bony deformities, Anorectal malformations or Arterial anomalies, and Rectal anomalies [LUMBAR] syndrome).[19,20] They can also ulcerate dramatically even before or in the absence of further proliferation. Differentiating capillary malformations from abortive hemangiomas/IHMAG can be challenging but observing telangiectatic blood vessels and a rim of pallor suggests an abortive hemangioma more so than a capillary malformation that tends to have more uniform color and no proliferative components. Unfortunately, the capillary malformations (which are actually nascent arteriovenous malformations) in capillary malformation-*arteriovenous malformation* (CM-AVM) syndrome typically also have a rim of vasoconstriction but they tend to have fewer telangiectasias.[21]

Therapy for hemangiomas should be based on preserving function and ensuring the best cosmetic result. Hemangiomas that affect vision, breathing, urination, and defecation or are in areas likely to ulcerate such as perineal or perioral usually require systemic therapy. In addition, hemangiomas on the head and neck or other cosmetically sensitive areas should be considered for therapy even if small. To decide how aggressive to be with therapy (oral or topical, laser or not), it is vital to try to predict what the skin will look like after the hemangioma has regressed. Deep hemangiomas and those with a gentle slope tend to have the best final look after involution, although any hemangioma on the central cheek or forehead can disrupt the elasticity and turgor of the skin, resulting in permanent wrinkling/atrophic scar. Hemangiomas with a very sharp angle at the skin surface (picture a mushroom cap) will often leave significant excess skin after involution that may require plastic surgical revision. Pedunculated hemangiomas also may ulcerate more easily if rapidly growing. A white, devascularized appearance at the center of a hemangioma often portends ulceration.[22] Ulcerated hemangiomas typically do not bleed excessively but one of the exceptions is scalp lesions. Ulcerations in the scalp can ulcerate through the skin into the scalp arteries and bleed extensively and should be treated more aggressively.

Timolol is off label but extremely effective at targeting the superficial aspect of hemangiomas.[23] The main benefit of timolol is as a proliferation preventative for small superficial or very early phase hemangiomas and for ulcerated hemangiomas (off label). Timolol is a potent β-blocker, and class-based risks including hypotension,

bradycardia, and hypoglycemia are possible but rare, given the low volume used. Caution is advised while using timolol in high blood flow areas (due to risk of increase absorption) such as the scalp, mucosa, and in ulcerated lesions but it can be very effective and is often used in all of these locations.[24] Timolol is usually started twice a day but many advocate for use three times a day. I usually advise the same precautions as taken with oral β-blockers including making sure the child has eaten before applying the timolol.

The main limiting factor to use of propranolol is usually sleep disturbance such as restless sleep or night terrors. There are a few ways to combat this. The doses are ideally split twice a day by about 10 hours, and the medicine peaks around 3 to 4 hours after the dose. Thus, if the first dose is given at 7 AM, the next can be at 5 PM, and the dose is mostly worn off by the time the children are sleeping. In addition, the AM and PM doses can be altered to give a lower dose in the evening; this may alter the efficacy and increase the risk of side effects but it may be better than not treating at all. Alternatively, atenolol or another β-blocker that does not cross the blood-brain barrier could be given.[25] These β-blockers are off label, and dosing guidelines and risks have not been formally established in this group but the effect on sleep may be less.

Capillary Malformations

Many vascular anomalies and related syndromes have been shown to be caused by mutations in genes involved in pathways guiding growth and division of cells. Many of these mutations are post-zygotic somatic mutations and thus may not be detected in tests using serum or saliva. Biopsy of the affected tissue is usually necessary to identify the causative gene. Differentiating the appearance of the various capillary malformations is key to recognizing with which syndrome they may be associated. The capillary malformations that are typically associated with Klippel-Trenaunay syndrome are usually dark purple and geometric with small purple papules that develop within them. The capillary malformations of CM-AVM syndrome tend to look as a pink macule, similar to a café au lait or thumb print, but have a rim of pallor around them.[26]

Skin of Color

It is extremely important to recognize the differences in presentation of skin conditions based on the relative amounts of melanin in the skin (see Okoji and colleagues' article, "Presentation of Common Skin Disorders in Pediatric Patients with Skin of Color," in this issue). For instance, a nevus sebaceous that is bright yellow in someone with very little melanin may seem more red or tan or hyperpigmented in someone with more melanin. Hemangiomas are similarly more hyperpigmented and do not display the same red color in someone with darker basal skin tones. Nevi will also be much darker in patients who have significantly more melanin. Nevi are similarly much lighter in patients who have very little melanin, making them very difficult to differentiate from Spitz nevi. Therefore, the history is extremely important when differentiating birthmarks. For instance, the look of a juvenile xanthogranuloma and an infantile hemangioma in a patient with skin of color can be very similar. Hemangiomas will not be fully formed at birth and will have a growth and then plateau and regression phases, which is different than the history of a juvenile xanthogranuloma. Therefore, history is critical and will help differentiate and diagnose when morphology fails.

The clinical appearance of inflammatory conditions also may be different in skin of color. AD in children with skin of color will often have more prominent follicular accentuation, which is accompanied by extreme itch and may need more aggressive therapy. There is also more postinflammatory hyperpigmentation on resolution of AD patches that may be overtreated due to the misunderstanding that the pigmentation is active disease. Alternatively, patients with very little melanin in their skin will often get red extremely easily on simple rubbing or touching in the absence of true dermatographism.

Many dermatitidis resolve with hyperpigmentation, and often parents will misperceive that the primary eruption is still active because the color change persists. As an example, in AD, it is important to educate parents to only actively treat the skin disease that is still red, inflamed, or papular and switch to maintenance phase when the skin is just hyperpigmented. Alternatively, postinflammatory hypopigmentation (PIH) happens naturally in AD, and parents will often mistakenly think that the topical steroids caused the PIH and thus inappropriately limit the amount of steroid they use. Education for these points is key.

Self-induced Skin Disorders

One of the most challenging sets of pediatric dermatologic conditions are those that are self-induced. Young children will often twirl or pick their skin as a coping method for anxiety or a way of self-soothing. Even when very apparent, parents sometimes have difficulty understanding or accepting that their children's habits are leading to their own alopecia or erosions. The parents of anxious children may also have similar traits because as a psychologist once told me "apple trees make apples."

Older children and adolescents may not admit to trichotillosis, lip licking, or nail picking. I find that the introduction of judgment in history taking is usually counterproductive. Instead of asking "are you licking your lips" or "rubbing your knuckles" (for instance), asking in an interested and almost supportive way such as "can you show me how you lick your lips" or "show me how you rub your knuckles" will often lead to a willing participant who demonstrates their habit, and this is often a revelation for the parents. In my own family, my daughter had a clear horizontal crease on her nose, which we often associate with the "allergic salute" although I had never seen her rub her nose. When I asked her to show me how she rubbed her nose, she immediately demonstrated the habit. So even transverse nasal creases can be due to a behavioral habit and not what we might otherwise associate it with. Similarly, hair pulling in kids is often self-soothing and may not be a psychiatric diagnosis or compulsive trait. This finding should prompt nuanced and nonjudgmental questions about the psychological and physical safety of the home and other environments. The parents should be reminded that these are not "bad behaviors" to be disciplined but rather just habits, sometimes done subconsciously, which require support and understanding to help break.

That said, some children do suffer from compulsive and other disorders and require proactive treatment. Oral N-acetylcysteine (NAC) was found to be effective for trichotillomania (trichotillosis) in a randomized controlled trial.[27] Since then it has been proposed for other obsessive compulsive/anxiety-related habits such as nail biting, skin picking, and rubbing the nails, leading to a habit tick deformity.[28] Acne excoriée is caused by incessant picking or popping of acne lesions leading to pigmentation and scarring. It can be challenging to diagnose the precise subtype of acne and properly treat, as scarring usually dominates the clinical picture. Along with traditional acne therapy, NAC can help decrease this habitual activity. There are no clear dosing guidelines for children. The pills taste like rotten eggs so it is hard to hide the smell if not swallowed.

Procedures

Procedures in children can be challenging for multiple reasons. There are a few tips and tricks that can make bedside procedures feasible, successful, and less intimidating and nontraumatic (for patients and parents alike). The most important initial consideration for pediatric procedures is positioning of the patient. Being held down while lying down can be terrifying. If possible, having young children sit up, sit in the lap of, or lie next to a parent or guardian is more comforting. Distraction is also very helpful, and offering videos, books, and video games and letting the child decide can optimize distraction.

Injections can be painful so buffering lidocaine with bicarbonate can help lessen the burning from the medication. I don't tell children "this won't hurt" or "you won't feel anything." If they are told this and then they feel anything at all, even if not painful, they may become very anxious. What I do to help younger kids feel more comfortable is gently gather the skin between the index and thumb (in a pinching position without hurting); this helps tent up the skin, and the slight pressure dampens the nerves. Also, when injecting, I usually say "you will feel my fingers pinching your skin." This type of gentle pinching is acceptable to children. When they feel the pinch of the needle, the younger children often perceive this as the pinch of my fingers and are less anxious.

Other ways to make the actual injection less painful include various ways of tricking the nerves into feeling different sensations or nothing. Cold sprays or cold packs before injection can help. There are various vibration tools such as proprietary vibrating devices that can help decrease the pain of procedures. The vibration overwhelms the ability of the nerves to conduct pain. It is also imperative, even if the child knows it is coming, to hide the actual needle so this does not induce a fight or flight response.

COMPLIANCE/ADHERENCE

Young children typically have built-in compliance managers because parents are usually very motivated to help their children. Teenagers, on the other hand, are usually somewhat independent in their skin care and often reluctant to listen to authority. There are a few ways of motivating teens that I have found successful:

- Try not to gang up on teens. They already recoil from being told what to do and if we act as agents of their parent's control, they will revolt. If a parent says "she never moisturizes even when I tell her to," a response directed at the child that also shames them is rarely productive.
- Address the child directly instead of only going through their parents.
- Ask them a little bit about their life to show that you are invested in them.

- Try to appeal to the child's motivations.
  - The teen may not want to use thick moisturizer because they don't want to look shiny at school. Options: offer them cream or once daily medication at night.
- Help them try to look into the future to see the benefits. If it is November you could say: "If you start using your retinoid now, in 2 months you will see a huge benefit so your acne will look much more clear by New Years!"

SUMMARY

Pediatric dermatology is an incredibly rewarding field. Children are resilient and funny and just want to know that you are advocating for their best interests. Teaming up with children and their parents can lead to fantastic therapeutic alliances and success. It is hoped that a few tips and pearls as described herein will help at the bedside and beyond.

CLINICS CARE POINTS

- Lanolin or methylisothiazolinone may be in mois- turizers or soaps therapeutic benefit of a particular medication needs to be balanced with the frequency of blood draws and injection molluscum can also present as cysts, inflamed papules, pustules, and abscesses.
- There are some variants of hemangiomas 396 including abortive hemangiomas or infantile hem- 397 angiomas with minimal or arrested growth 398 (IHMAG), which are telangiectatic patches often 399 present at birth with a rim of vasoconstriction.
- Differentiating the appearance of the various capillary malformations is key to recognizing with which syndrome they may be associated.
- It is extremely important to recognize the differ- ences in presentation of skin conditions based on the relative amounts of melanin in the skin.

DISCLOSURE

Dr James Treat is a consultant for Palvella, INC.

REFERENCES

1. Dhingra N, Gulati N, Guttman-Yassky E. Mechanisms of contact sensitization offer insights into the role of barrier defects vs. intrinsic immune

abnormalities as drivers of atopic dermatitis. J Invest Dermatol 2013;133(10):2311–4.

2. Williams HC. Twice-weekly topical corticosteroid therapy may reduce atopic dermatitis relapses. Arch Dermatol 2004;140(9):1151–2.

3. Owen JL, Vakharia PP, Silverberg JI. The role and diagnosis of allergic contact dermatitis in patients with atopic dermatitis. Am J Clin Dermatol 2018; 19(3):293–302.

4. Towell AM, Feuillie C, Vitry P, et al. Staphylococcus aureus binds to the N-terminal region of corneodesmosin to adhere to the stratum corneum in atopic dermatitis. Proc Natl Acad Sci 2021;118(1). e2014444118.

5. Huang JT, Rademaker A, Paller AS. Dilute bleach baths for Staphylococcus aureus colonization in atopic dermatitis to decrease disease severity. Arch Dermatol 2011;147(2):246–7.

6. Chamlin SL, Mattson CL, Frieden IJ, et al. The price of pruritus: sleep disturbance and cosleeping in atopic dermatitis. Arch Pediatr Adolesc Med 2005; 159(8):745–50.

7. Bikowski J. Barrier disease beyond eczema: management of juvenile plantar dermatosis. Pract Dermatol Pediatr 2010;28–31.

8. Stefanaki C, Lagogianni E, Kontochristopoulos G, et al. Psoriasis in children: a retrospective analysis. J Eur Acad Dermatol Venereol 2011;25(4):417–21.

9. Mercy K, Kwasny M, Cordoro KM, et al. Clinical manifestations of pediatric psoriasis: results of a multicenter study in the United States. Pediatr Dermatol 2013;30(4):424–8.

10. Popadic S, Nikolic M. Pustular psoriasis in childhood and adolescence: a 20-year single-center experience. Pediatr Dermatol 2014;31(5):575–9.

11. Meza-Romero R, Navarrete-Dechent C, Downey C. Molluscum contagiosum: an update and review of new perspectives in etiology, diagnosis, and treatment. Clin Cosmet Investig Dermatol 2019;12:373.

12. Silverberg NB. Molluscum contagiosum virus infection can trigger atopic dermatitis disease onset or flare. Cutis 2018;102(3):191–4.

13. Berger EM, Orlow SJ, Patel RR, et al. Experience with molluscum contagiosum and associated inflammatory reactions in a pediatric dermatology practice: the bump that rashes. Arch Dermatol 2012; 148(11):1257–64.

14. Scheinfeld N. Treatment of molluscum contagiosum a brief review and discussion of a case successfully treated with adapelene. Dermatol Online J 2007; 13(3):15.

15. Alikhan A, Griffin JR, Newman CC. Use of Candida antigen injections for the treatment of verruca vulgaris: A two-year mayo clinic experience. J Dermatol Treat 2016;27(4):355–8.

16. Nickles MA, Sergeyenko A, Bain M. Treatment of warts with topical cidofovir in a pediatric patient. Dermatol Online J 2019;25(5). 13030/qt5sq5b24g.

17. Gladsjo JA, Alió Sáenz AB, Bergman J, et al. 5% 5-Fluorouracil cream for treatment of verruca vulgaris in children. Pediatr Dermatol 2009;26(3):279–85.

18. Suh KY, Frieden IJ. Infantile hemangiomas with minimal or arrested growth: a retrospective case series. Arch Dermatol 2010;146(9):971–6.

19. Metry D, Heyer G, Hess C, et al. Consensus statement on diagnostic criteria for PHACE syndrome. Pediatrics 2009;124(5):1447–56.

20. Iacobas I, Burrows PE, Frieden IJ, et al. LUMBAR: association between cutaneous infantile hemangiomas of the lower body and regional congenital anomalies. J Pediatr 2010;157(5):795–801.

21. Iznardo H, Roé E, Puig L, et al. Good response to pulsed dye laser in patients with capillary malformation-arteriovenous malformation syndrome (CM-AVM). Pediatr Dermatol 2020;37(2):342–4.

22. Maguiness SM, Hoffman WY, McCalmont TH, et al. Early white discoloration of infantile hemangioma: a sign of impending ulceration. Arch Dermatol 2010; 146(11):1235–9.

23. Pope E, Chakkittakandiyil A. Topical timolol gel for infantile hemangiomas: a pilot study. Arch Dermatol 2010;146(5):564–5.

24. Weibel L, Barysch MJ, Scheer HS, et al. Topical timolol for infantile hemangiomas: evidence for efficacy and degree of systemic absorption. Pediatr Dermatol 2016;33(2):184–90.

25. Villalba-Moreno AM, Cotrina-Luque J, Del Vayo-Benito CA, et al. Nadolol for the treatment of infantile hemangioma. Am J Health-System Pharm 2015; 72(1):44–6.

26. Rozas-Muñoz E, Frieden IJ, Roé E, et al. Vascular stains: proposal for a clinical classification to improve diagnosis and management. Pediatr Dermatol 2016;33(6):570–84.

27. Grant JE, Odlaug BL, Kim SW. N-acetylcysteine, a glutamate modulator, in the treatment of trichotillomania: a double-blind, placebo-controlled study. Arch Gen Psychiatry 2009;66(7):756–63.

28. Grant JE, Chamberlain SR, Redden SA, et al. N-acetylcysteine in the treatment of excoriation disorder: a randomized clinical trial. JAMA psychiatry 2016; 73(5):490–6.

Towards a More Inclusive Environment in the Dermatology Clinic

An Introduction to Using Thoughtful Language in the Practice of Dermatology

Michael Barton, MD, Markus D. Boos, MD, PhD*

KEYWORDS

- Language • Diversity • Inclusivity • Patient-centered care • Stigma

KEY POINTS

- The specific language used to interact with patients and colleagues can directly influence thought and perception.
- Adopting a patient-centered, inclusive dermatologic vernacular conveys respect, accounts for differences, and promotes equity.
- Language evolves over time and so must our ability to relinquish outdated and offensive terminology from our specialty's vocabulary.
- Shifting from inaccurate, nondescriptive diagnoses toward neutral terminology that reflects pathophysiology may help facilitate more patient-centered nomenclature in dermatology.

INTRODUCTION

Language is a singular method of expression and communication, having been referred to as "one of the most exquisitely sophisticated and powerful products of the human mind."[1] Within dermatology, a specific vernacular allows providers to quickly communicate a particular diagnosis via precise morphologic descriptions (eg, "grouped vesicles on an erythematous base" to describe a herpes simplex virus infection), or evocative imagery ("islands in a sea of fire" to refer to the morbilliform eruption of dengue). Learning the "language of dermatology" and subsequently using it appropriately is thus a central component of training in our discipline.

Nevertheless, language is more than just a manner of conveying thought; it also *influences* thought and perception.[1] As a result, the words that we use to describe medical conditions and a patient's experience with these conditions impact how we view those who seek dermatologic care, how we deliver this care, and subsequent patient perceptions of the quality of care they receive. Specifically, language can be used to positively frame perspectives on medical conditions and their treatment, in turn strengthening therapeutic relationships and giving patients a sense of confidence and agency. Wielded unartfully, however, language can also marginalize, stigmatize, and engender feelings of doubt and shame, with negative health outcomes.[2] Thoughtful employment of language has been identified as important for maintaining the *accuracy* of information provided, preventing *power* imbalances, *labeling* individuals, *framing* an individual's experience of their condition, and preventing *stereotyping*.[2] In this review, we seek to highlight ways in which pediatric and adult dermatologists can incorporate thoughtful language that is patient-centered and inclusive, to improve the quality of patient care.

Division of Dermatology, Department of Pediatrics, University of Washington School of Medicine, Seattle Children's Hospital, 4800 Sand Point Way Northeast, OC.9.833, Seattle, WA 98105, USA
* Corresponding author.
E-mail address: markus.boos@seattlechildrens.org

Dermatol Clin 40 (2022) 103–108
https://doi.org/10.1016/j.det.2021.09.008
0733-8635/22/© 2021 Elsevier Inc. All rights reserved.

A PATIENT-CENTERED APPROACH TO LANGUAGE

The Linguistic Society of America defines inclusive language as "language that acknowledges diversity, conveys respect to all people, is sensitive to differences, and promotes equal opportunities."[3] Nevertheless, putting this into practice can be a challenge, because individuals may receive the same language differently depending on various aspects of their identity and culture; an individual's attitude toward the same words may even change with time.[2,4] In general, use of person-centered language is recommended during patient care. Person-centered language prioritizes an individual's agency to self-identify as they choose and, in the context of medical care, avoids labeling an individual as their medical condition. As such, person-centered language is a means by which providers can display respect and create a safe clinic environment.[4]

Use of Inclusive Language when Addressing and Identifying the Patient

The American Medical Association Code of Medical Ethics states that "the relationship between a patient and a physician is based on trust, which gives rise to physicians' ethical responsibility to place patients' welfare above the physician's own self-interest...and to advocate for their patients' welfare."[5] Use of inclusive, patient-centered language may help to engender this trust, and this process can begin as early as during introductions at an initial clinic visit. Specifically, providers should be mindful of patients' inherent rights to self-determination and self-identification and enquire about an individual's name and pronouns accordingly. This method is particularly vital when caring for transgender, agender, gender diverse, 2-spirit, or other sexual and gender minority (SGM) youth whose gender identity exists outside of a traditional "female-male" binary.[6,7] These children may use gender-neutral pronouns such as "they/them/theirs," "ze/hir/hirs," or other variations.[6] Not assuming a patient's gender and asking questions with the use of gender-neutral language until the patient's name and pronouns can be elicited are meaningful ways to support individuals' rights to self-identify, provide patient comfort, and build strong therapeutic alliances.[8] In general, we recommend using the same terms that a patient uses when referring to themselves, their loved ones, and their relationships.[7,9] Moreover, repeated misuse of a patient's stated name or pronoun can lead to distress, in turn damaging the doctor-patient relationship and perpetuating health care disparities that exist for SGM youth.[8,10]

A recent review in the *Journal of the American Academy of Dermatology* provides more extensive recommendations and specific examples for using inclusive language when caring for SGM individuals; these principles, as well as examples of inclusive language, are summarized in **Box 1**.[9]

Patient Labels

Providers' choice of words when referring to and discussing patients also carries important implications for care. Specifically, Fleitas[11] argues that when providers label patients by their medical condition (ie, "The Atopics on my schedule," "The flaring Psoriatic in the ED"), it increases the risk that these individuals will be dehumanized and seen as a disease state rather than as children with unique identities; this in turn may influence the quality of care they receive. Furthermore, referring to individuals in this way incorporates medical pathology as the essential quality of their identity, instead of one of many aspects of it.[2,12] Although a certain convenience exists for health care providers when using such labels, it is important to ask: at what cost? Labeling and defining children

---

Box 1
Inclusive, gender-neutral language to use during the patient visit[6,7,9]

General principles

- Do not make assumptions about a patient's gender or pronouns.
- Use gender-neutral terminology ("they," "you") until the patient's name and pronouns can be elicited. Avoid use of the term "it," which is considered dehumanizing and offensive.
- Allow the patient to express the terms they use for their loved ones and relationships and respond by using those same terms (ie, "boyfriend," "girlfriend," "partner").

Examples of inclusive language

- "We want to make sure that our clinic is a safe space for all of our patients, so we ask everyone what their name and pronouns are."
- "What name should I use when talking to you?"
- "Which pronouns should I use when addressing you: he, she, they, something else, or none at all?"
- "Are you in a relationship?"
- "Who is joining you during our clinic visit today?"

as their medical condition may prevent providers from seeing them as anything more; when such labels are overheard by the patient, this can lead to distress, lowered self-esteem, and mistrust of medical care.[11] Instead, providers should be mindful to use person-first language that emphasizes the individual and not their medical condition (ie, "Jane is in the ED with a psoriasis flare"), in an effort to reduce stereotype and biases.[13] Use of such patient-centered language in turn empowers children to see their condition as a manageable part of their overall health, and not a disease that defines them.

CULTURAL MINDFULNESS AND DERMATOLOGIC DISEASE
The Naming of Dermatologic Conditions

The vernacular we use as dermatologists is fraught with diagnoses that unintentionally leave patients and their families feeling marginalized, offended, misrepresented, or stereotyped. If the goals of inclusive language include conveying respect to all patients and practicing awareness and responsiveness to differences, then certain diagnoses that unfairly emphasize or denigrate race and gender or assign culpability based on these personal characteristics must be avoided. Before considering select examples of these diagnoses and their proposed alternatives, it is important to acknowledge that as language evolves, terms that were previously used in a given place and time can eventually acquire drastically different connotations. Importantly, using inclusive language extends beyond its use with patients; it must be incorporated into how we communicate with colleagues, publish articles, and even report data.[14]

Congenital dermal melanocytosis (CDM) is an often spontaneously resolving birthmark commonly located on the lumbosacral region of newborns and characterized morphologically by nonpalpable, blue to slate-gray patches. Although its prevalence is greater in newborns with darker skin tones, it has no absolute predilection for one specific race or ethnicity. Despite this fact, CDM has historically been referred to as *Mongolian spots* by clinicians and families. Although the formal clinical term *congenital dermal melanocytosis* has been increasingly adopted over time, its historical title continues to be widely referenced by numerous primary and specialty providers, families, and authors.

To better understand the negative, racist connotation of the term Mongolian spot, a historic understanding of racial categorization at the time this term was coined must be briefly reviewed.[15] In the late eighteenth century, the Western concept of race was heavily influenced by German physician and anthropologist Johann Blumenbach, who believed that individuals could be categorized into 5 different races based on variations in phenotype, including skin color.[16] Others at the time adopted this classification scheme of race, with some distorting their view of white individuals (referred to at the time as Caucasian) as superior to others.[17] Unfortunately, the "Mongolian race," denoted by Blumenbach and other anthropologists of his time as primarily populations living in East Asia, were denigrated in this racist, hierarchical categorization, being described as having "weaker bodies," "natural cowardliness," "extraordinary excitability," and "lack of ability to work hard."[18] When what we now term CDM was first reported in the Western medical literature, this cutaneous finding was proclaimed to be a distinct racial characteristic of the Mongols.[19] Theories circulated, with some hypothesizing that Mongolian spots/CDM may represent a physical reversion to an ancestral cutaneous state, implying that newborns harboring these birthmarks were more primitive than other races perceived to be more advanced.[20] Unfortunately, over time individuals with chromosomal aberrancies and developmental delay were often described as having "mongoloid" features.[21] The imprecise terminology used to describe these common birthmarks subsequently became associated with racial inferiority and genetic syndromes. Taking this background into consideration, it becomes clear why the descriptive, culturally responsive terminology of "congenital dermal melanocytosis" is recommended.

Vancomycin-induced red man syndrome is another diagnosis with dermatologic manifestations that invokes a racist stereotype. This histamine-mediated reaction that results in erythema and pruritus, most commonly of the face and upper body, often occurs secondary to rapid infusion of vancomycin. Initially described in 1959 as "an anaphylactoid reaction to vancomycin," this condition assumed its more common and racially insensitive title in 1985 after a publication described it in the *New England Journal of Medicine*.[22,23] The terms "redskin" or "red man" are contemptuous, racist slurs first uttered in the seventeenth century to describe American Indian or Indigenous peoples. The continued use of these terms in medical vernacular demonstrates an ongoing lack of awareness and sensitivity toward this historically and persistently exploited population. Recent directives have been proposed to modify the naming of this diagnosis back to its original, more informative title, "vancomycin flushing reaction," which more closely associates with the pathophysiology of the phenomenon and avoids race-based diagnosis.[24]

The implementation of inclusive language attempts to advance our communication beyond use of racialized, and often racist, generalizations. Such language no longer conflates race with a disease state, when in actuality, the disease itself exists independent of race. Closely identifying a specific population with a specific medical condition or diagnosis risks insinuating that there is something inherently inferior about these populations and activates our own, often unrecognized, implicit biases. By replacing potentially offensive and inaccurate diagnoses with their more edifying and descriptive titles such as "congenital dermal melanocytosis" and "vancomycin flushing reaction" we embrace a medical vernacular that displays respect, inclusion, and knowledge.

Stigmatization and "the Blame Game"

Despite the efforts made toward accepting and normalizing disorders of mental health, there are few areas in medicine and society as stigmatizing as psychiatric disorders. Dermatology often interfaces with mental health, and several psychocutaneous disorders possess names that pose a risk to further insult and stigmatize patients. Diagnoses such as "trichotillomania," "delusions of parasitosis," and "neurotic excoriations" are often perceived as judgmental by patients and evoke resistance and denial, which only hinders the patient-provider relationship and interferes with therapeutic considerations and compliance.[25] With patients' increased access to electronic medical records, it is important to remain transparent and factual, but implicating that patients are maniacal, delusional, or neurotic in writing is even less likely to foster a congruent partnership moving forward. Shifting away from insensitive language with objectionable connotations and adopting neutral, patient-centered nomenclature may diminish barriers during an already challenging encounter. "Neuromechanical alopecia," "trichotillosis," "pseudoparasitic dysaesthesia," and simply "excoriations" are proposed modifications to help facilitate a more trusting doctor-patient relationship.[25]

Medical conditions that are most often stigmatized share 2 essential qualities: individuals with these conditions are perceived as being at fault for acquiring them, as well as possessing a significant amount of control over choices that influence the severity and course of the condition.[26] However, these assumptions are often inaccurate. Take, for example, a child with a slower rate of weight gain in childhood than expected for age and sex, previously known as "failure to thrive." This outmoded term inappropriately blames the child or their parents for growing more slowly than expected, for reasons that may be beyond their control. As such, the term "faltering growth" is now preferred by most organizations, because periods of slow growth may represent transient, blameless, and uncontrollable variation from expected patterns. Moreover, the word "failure" may be perceived as pejorative by families.[27] Slight alterations to the words we use when communicating with families can reduce the stigma, guilt, and blame surrounding specific diagnoses and may have a tremendous capacity to shift perceptions and relieve feelings of helplessness or despair. Ultimately, use of inclusive language cultivates support and acceptance and empowers patients to have a sense of optimism and control over their medical condition.

Use of Eponyms in Dermatology

Eponyms are commonly used in dermatology to pay homage toward individuals and reflect on the rich history associated with dermatologic conditions (Sweet syndrome), diagnostic criteria (Hanifin and Rajka), and various related discoveries (Koebner and Wolf phenomena).[28] It is often suggested that the use of eponyms is becoming less frequent; however, their use in the medical literature remains common.[29] Proponents for the continued use of eponyms argue that these illustrious titles often have concise communicative roles that allow providers to "enrich our language and to honor the legacy of those dedicated souls who have catapulted our specialty to amazing heights."[28,30] Unfortunately, the individuals enshrined by these eponyms may also be connected to horrific events in human history, which makes honoring them inappropriate and offensive (eg, Dr Friedrich Wegener's affiliation with the Nazi party before and after World War II). In addition to Wegener granulomatosis (now referred to as "granulomatosis with polyangiitis"), Reiter syndrome (now referred to as "reactive arthritis") is another eponymous diagnosis that has fallen out of favor given its association with a Nazi physician who committed war crimes. Although professional societies have recommended replacing eponymous diagnoses with terminology more appropriately rooted in pathophysiology, downstream adoption of such changes may be inconsistent and the resultant rebranding often leaves providers and patients alike confused.[31] As such, it is important to thoughtfully assess the benefits gained by using newer, neutral, but often

Table 1
Suggested terms for specific dermatologic conditions with outdated or culturally insensitive names

Historic Nomenclature	Proposed Alternatives
Mongolian spots	Congenital dermal melanocytosis
Red man syndrome	Vancomycin flushing reaction
Trichotillomania	Neuromechanical alopecia/trichotillosis
Delusions of parasitosis	Pseudoparasitic dysaesthesia
Neurotic excoriations	Excoriations
Failure to thrive	Faltering growth
Wegener granulomatosis	Granulomatosis with polyangiitis
Reiter syndrome	Reactive arthritis

unfamiliar terms in discussion with patients and colleagues; there may be situations in which a specific eponym lacks a negative association and may be considered more patient-centered than the alternative (eg, a patient may be more likely to remember that they have been diagnosed with Sweet syndrome rather than the linguistically cumbersome "acute febrile neutrophilic dermatosis"). Nevertheless, we recommend avoiding use of eponyms as much as possible and encourage patient education about the reasons for diagnostic name changes as appropriate. Particularly for patients and families who have been harmed by the historic terms discussed herein, an honest acknowledgment and transparent discussion about the role that medicine has played in perpetuating societal inequities and our efforts to counter them may improve patient trust and strengthen the doctor-patient relationship. **Table 1** provides a select list of eponyms and other diagnostic terms commonly used in dermatology, with recommended alternate nomenclature.

SUMMARY

Language is an essential aspect of the patient-provider relationship. Language is used to help establish rapport and plays a pivotal role in relaying diagnostic, prognostic, and therapeutic information. Incorporating thoughtful, patient-centered, and inclusive language into our verbal and written communication has the potential to build trust and create a safer environment for our patients and their families. This process starts with the patient introduction and prioritizes use of appropriate, patient-identifying pronouns; it continues by avoiding the labeling of individuals as their medical condition and emphasizing a patient-first mindset. Inclusive language refrains from unnecessarily attaching race or gender to a

diagnosis and denounces the placement of unfair blame on others. Finally, it attempts to communicate in a succinct and clear manner, which may be facilitated by using understandable, pathophysiology-derived terminology. Although not intended to be an exhaustive list, this review highlights select aspects of communication that create a supportive environment for patients and their families.

CLINICS CARE POINTS

- The language used to describe medical conditions and a patient's experience with these conditions impact how we view those who seek dermatologic care, how we deliver this care, and subsequent patient perceptions of the quality of care they receive.

- Adopting a patient-centered, inclusive vernacular conveys respect, builds trust between physician and patient, accounts for individual differences and promotes equity.

- Shifting from inaccurate, non-descriptive diagnoses towards neutral terminology that reflects pathophysiology may help facilitate more patient-centered nomenclature in dermatology.

DISCLOSURE/ CONFLICTS OF INTEREST

The authors of this article have nothing to disclose.

ACKNOWLEDGMENTS

The authors would like to thank Shaquita Bell, MD, and Alicia Adiele for their thoughtful review and comments on this article.

REFERENCES

1. Thierry G. Neurolinguistic relativity: how language flexes human perception and cognition. Lang Learn 2016;66:690–713.
2. Banasiak K, Cleary D, Bajurny V, et al. Language matters - a diabetes Canada consensus statement. Can J Diabetes 2020;44:370–3.
3. LSA Executive Committee. Linguistic Society of America Guidelines for Inclusive language. Available at: https://www.linguisticsociety.org/sites/default/files/Inclusive_Lg_Guidelines.pdf.
4. Counseling@Northwestern, the Online Master of Arts in Counseling program from The Family Institute at Northwestern University. Inclusive Language Guide. Available at: https://counseling.northwestern.edu/blog/inclusive-language-guide/.
5. American Medical Association. Patient-physician relationships. Available at: https://www.ama-assn.org/delivering-care/ethics/patient-physician-relationships.
6. Liszewski W, Peebles JK, Yeung H, et al. Persons of nonbinary gender - awareness, visibility, and health disparities. N Engl J Med 2018;379:2391–3.
7. Boos MD, Yeung H, Inwards-Breland D. Dermatologic care of sexual and gender minority/LGBTQIA youth, Part I: an update for the dermatologist on providing inclusive care. Pediatr Dermatol 2019;36:581–6.
8. Gridley SJ, Crouch JM, Evans Y, et al. Youth and caregiver perspectives on barriers to gender-affirming health care for transgender youth. J Adolesc Health 2016;59:254–61.
9. Yeung H, Luk KM, Chen SC, et al. Dermatologic care for lesbian, gay, bisexual, and transgender persons: terminology, demographics, health disparities, and approaches to care. J Am Acad Dermatol 2019;80:581–9.
10. Steever J, Francis J, Gordon LP, et al. Sexual minority youth. Prim Care 2014;41:651–69.
11. Fleitas J. The power of words: examining the linguistic landscape of pediatric nursing. MCN Am J Matern Child Nurs 2003;28:384–8 [quiz 389–90].
12. Fleischman S. I am ... , I have ... , I suffer from ... : a linguist reflects on the language of illness and disease. J Med Humanit 1999;20:3–32.
13. Dickinson JK, Guzman SJ, Maryniuk MD, et al. The use of language in diabetes care and education. Diabetes Care 2017;40:1790–9.
14. Baeckens S, Blomberg SP, Shine R. Inclusive science: ditch insensitive terminology. Nature 2020;580:185.
15. Zhong CS, Huang JT, Nambudiri VE. Revisiting the history of the 'Mongolian spot': the background and implications of a medical term used today. Pediatr Dermatol 2019;36:755–7.
16. Blumenbach JF. The Anthropological treatises of Johann friedrich Blumenbach. London: Anthropological Society; 1865.
17. Temkin O. German concepts of ontogeny and history around 1800. Bull Hist Med 1950;24:227–46.
18. Race and racism in modern East Asia: western and eastern constructions. Brill; 2014.
19. Baelz, E. Die Korperlichen Eigenschafter de Japaner. Mitt. Deutsch. Ges. Natur u. Volkerk. Ostasiens 1885;4(40):35–103.
20. Ashley-Montagu MF. The concept of atavism. Science 1938;87:462–3.
21. Ward OC. John Langdon Down: the man and the message. Syndr Res Pract J Sarah Duffen Cent 1999;6:19–24.
22. Rothenberg HJ. Anaphylactoid reaction to vancomycin. J Am Med Assoc 1959;171:1101–2.
23. Garrelts JC, Peterie JD. Vancomycin and the 'red man's syndrome'. N Engl J Med 1985;312:245.
24. Austin JP, Foster BA, Empey A. Replace red man syndrome with vancomycin flushing reaction. Hosp Pediatr 2020;10:623–4.
25. Walling HW, Swick BL. Psychocutaneous syndromes: a call for revised nomenclature. Clin Exp Dermatol 2007;32:317–9.
26. SAMHSA'S Center for the Application of Prevention Technologies. Words matter: how language choice can reduce stigma 2017. Available at: http://www.wvha.org/getmedia/53991bb8-2978-4e38-a58e-10a9e3b6506e/SAMHSA_Words-Matter.pdf.aspx.
27. National Guideline Alliance (UK). Faltering Growth – recognition and management. Excellence (UK): National Institute for Health and Care; 2017.
28. Barankin B. Saving the eponym. Int J Dermatol 2005;44:134–5.
29. Thomas PB. Are medical eponyms really dying out? A study of their usage in the historical biomedical literature. J R Coll Physicians Edinb 2016;46:295–9.
30. Canziani T. The status of medical eponyms: advantages and disadvantages. In: Teaching medical English: methods and models 2011;. p. 217–30.
31. Falk RJ, Gross WL, Guillevin L, et al. Granulomatosis with polyangiitis (Wegener's): an alternative name for Wegener's granulomatosis. J Am Soc Nephrol 2011;22:587–8.

Addressing Climate-Related Health Impacts During the Patient Encounter
A Practical Guide for Pediatric Dermatologists

Mary D. Sun, BSE, BA[a], Markus D. Boos, MD, PhD[b,c], Sarah J. Coates, MD[d],*

KEYWORDS

- Climate change • Social determinants of health • Pollution • History of present illness (HPI)
- Patient education • Narrative medicine • Motivational interviewing • Risk communication

KEY POINTS

- Pediatric populations are expected to bear the majority of climate change impacts, with racial minorities and children living in poorer countries being particularly vulnerable.
- Dermatologists should be aware of climate-sensitive health impacts and their intersections with social factors.
- Strategies including targeted risk communication, motivational interviewing, and storytelling can help facilitate climate discussions during the patient encounter.
- Specific additions can also be made to the medical and social history to elicit climate-sensitive health risks of pediatric patients.
- The authors summarize common dermatologic health impacts related to environmental exposures and provide sample scripts for climate messaging.

BACKGROUND
How Does Climate Change Affect Dermatologic Health in Pediatric Populations?

Climate change is increasingly recognized as an important factor in dermatologic health.[1,2] Climate impacts are particularly significant in pediatric populations, which are estimated to bear nearly 90% of the climate change disease burden and already account for a disproportionate share of preventable climate-related deaths.[3] Because of age-related physiology and developmental differences, children are often at higher risk for serious morbidity from environmental exposures. Higher temperatures correlate with pediatric emergency department visits not only for asthma exacerbations but also for heat stress, because children must divert more cardiac output to dissipate heat than adults.[3] The incidence of vector-borne diseases—such as cutaneous leishmaniasis, Dengue, and malaria—and diarrheal diseases, all of which present more severely in younger patients, is expected to increase with warming temperatures.[4,5]

Furthermore, early and chronic exposure to harmful environmental conditions can lead to adverse effects across the lifespan. Smoke from epidemic wildfires, particulate matter in greenhouse gas emissions, and ozone depletion

[a] Icahn School of Medicine at Mount Sinai, 1 Gustave Levy Pl, New York, NY 10025, USA; [b] University of Washington School of Medicine, Seattle, WA, USA; [c] Seattle Children's Hospital, 4800 Sand Point Way Northeast, Seattle, WA 98105, USA; [d] Department of Dermatology, The University of California, San Francisco, 1701 Divisadero Street Floor 3, San Francisco, CA 94115, USA
* Corresponding author.
E-mail address: sarah.coates@ucsf.edu

Dermatol Clin 40 (2022) 109–116
https://doi.org/10.1016/j.det.2021.09.007
0733-8635/22/© 2021 Elsevier Inc. All rights reserved.

contribute to increasing levels of ambient air pollution and the worst global air quality levels recorded in decades.[6,7] These pollutants can permanently affect the function of developing lungs and predispose to respiratory illness, increase antibiotic use in infants,[8] and cause or worsen inflammatory and atopic conditions. Large cohort studies have linked atopic dermatitis and acne prevalence to air pollution, as well as environmental exposures such as tobacco smoke and dust mites to the exacerbation of inflammatory dermatoses.[9] Climate change also leads to extreme weather fluctuations that can disrupt food supply systems and lead to food insecurity, negatively affecting childhood nutrition at times that are critical for growth and cognitive development.[4] Moreover, psychosocial stress, which often occurs during and after natural disasters, has also been linked to disease exacerbations in patients with atopic dermatitis, psoriasis, vitiligo, and alopecia areata.[10–13] The impacts of these and other climate-related health exposures lead to cumulative adverse health effects over time that may persist into adulthood.

Which Populations are Particularly Vulnerable?

As many health-related harms, experiences of climate change are mediated by social factors including systemic racism, poverty, and lack of access to health care. The unique dependence of children on their caregivers and communities contributes to higher climate-related vulnerabilities in certain pediatric populations. Non-White, Indigenous, and low-income communities suffer disproportionately from extreme weather events and exposure to small particulate matter from wildfires.[14–16] In the United States, racial minorities are also more likely to be burdened by rent or experience homelessness, worsening the health impacts of climate exposures.[17] Climate change also profoundly affects children in poorer countries, whose populations experience high rates of food and housing insecurity that are further amplified by natural disasters. Nearly 13 million children are displaced by natural disasters each year and become at-risk for physical trauma, abuse, mental health issues, inadequate access to quality health care, and waterborne and zoonotic infectious diseases.[3]

DISCUSSION
How Can Pediatric Dermatologists Address Climate Change in the Clinic?

Climate events and environmental exposures affect the presentation of inflammatory, infectious, and sun-related dermatoses. To safeguard the health of pediatric patients, dermatologists should be aware of climate-sensitive health impacts and their intersections with other social factors. In the following sections, the authors describe strategies that can help facilitate discussions about climate change and provide specific additions that can be made during the patient encounter to address climate-sensitive health risks. They also summarize common dermatologic health impacts related to environmental exposures and provide sample scripts for climate messaging.

Strategies for discussing climate-related topics
Given the potentially polarizing nature of this topic, pediatric dermatologists should take a nonjudgmental stance when discussing climate change with patients and their parents/guardians. In general, focusing on specific, actionable connections between environmental exposures and health consequences can be more effective than attempting to change personal viewpoints. The goal of these communications should be to comfortably engage parents/guardians so that they make educated and appropriate decisions regarding the care of their children. To this end, the authors identify several communication frameworks that can be useful in climate discussion scenarios and provide brief examples in **Table 1**.

- *Targeted risk communication:* the perception that climate change can drive adverse health outcomes including mortality, disease incidence, and lack of access to basic necessities has been strongly correlated with support for climate change mitigation policies.[18] As sources of trusted recommendations in an increasingly complex information environment, health care providers are uniquely situated to provide patients with credible resources regarding these and other health risks of climate change.[19] Oftentimes, patients may be unaware of the many ways in which they are stakeholders in their local and global environments. Developing a working knowledge of how patients and their families may already engage with climate information (eg, online videos, television shows, social media) can be particularly helpful, as additional context and reflective discussion can be provided during the clinical encounter.[20] A recent scoping review suggests that risk communication efforts are most effective during short-term extreme weather events, highlighting an important opportunity for proactive communication with patients living in high-risk areas or who have

Table 1
Brief examples of strategies used to frame climate discussions

Strategy	Example Scenario	Key Characteristics	Sample Framing
Targeted risk communication	Hurricane is expected to make landfall in a coastal city	• Consistent messaging • Clear information delivered in an accessible way • Unambiguous, action-oriented recommendations	"I want to make sure that you and your family know about Hurricane X and the latest recommendations from FEMA. Is there anything preventing you from evacuating by tomorrow night?"
Motivational interviewing	Urban-dwelling patient with asthma who spends most of the day playing outside	• Genuine interest in understanding and working from the patient's worldview • Reflective, open-ended questions • Affirming language	"It is clear you care a lot about your child's health. What do you and your family think of the air pollution and extreme heat and how that might affect her eczema and asthma?"
Storytelling	Patient with severe atopic dermatitis living in the Southeastern Mendocino Interior, an area prone to wildfires	• Fosters connectedness with patient and their community • Illustrates impact of specific climate factor • Empathetic language	"This situation reminds me of when our son's eczema got worse after the wildfires last fall. The smoke was hard to avoid, and I can imagine that seeing these eczema flares is tough on your family as well. I'd be happy to share some of the tools we used to track air quality and minimize the effects of indoor air pollution."

predisposing medical and/or social factors.[21] In emergency situations, providers should prioritize actionable information and encourage compliance with the most up-to-date safety recommendations.

• *Motivational interviewing:* motivational interviewing (MI) is an evidence-based approach structured as a series of brief dialogues. Instead of the clinician simply making recommendations to which the patient is expected to adhere, MI focuses on building rapport and understanding the patient's or parent/guardian's perspectives and motivations. The goal is to establish a partnership wherein the physician provides support and information when asked, which may be especially applicable in the case of medical issues

related to climate change.[22] Parents/guardians may be more interested in learning about direct health risks and available treatments than the systems-level nature of climate shifts. In MI encounters, parents/guardians should feel a sense of control that can ultimately be directed to motivate behavioral change. Importantly, providers can effectively implement MI without substantially extending the clinical encounter. MI has been used successfully for the management of dermatologic conditions including psoriasis and can be effectively implemented by a variety of medical professionals.[23–25] These techniques can be used to deliver consistent and compassionate messaging about actionable steps that patients and their families can take to combat health-related harms of climate change.

- *Storytelling:* there is growing evidence that the use of narrative frameworks can play a key role in facilitating productive conversations about climate change.[26] Human cognition is organized around narrative structures, and stories are therefore often more engaging, easier to comprehend, and more resonant with nonexpert audiences than traditional logic-oriented scientific communication.[27–29] By introducing or reframing social and cultural contexts that are relevant to the patient, clinicians can use narrative approaches to better navigate the complexities of climate change, sustainability practices, and intersecting social inequities.[30] Importantly, successful storytelling is predicated on first understanding the patient's own stories and beliefs about the urgency of and their role in climate change. How someone "stories" their own lived experiences is an important determinant of how they will receive and potentially adopt suggestions regarding adaptive climate behaviors—this can be especially crucial in the case of individuals who have experienced extreme weather events and climate migration.[31,32] To elicit information about additional medical, sociocultural, and institutional factors that may affect a patient's capacity for behavioral change, providers should use accessible language and ask open-ended questions during conversation.[28] In a storytelling model, both patient and provider engage in learning experiences to prompt reflection and rework knowledge of climate change.

Additions to the medical history

When taking a patient's medical history, several climate-focused additions can be made to aspects of the history of present illness. The goal of these additions is to develop an understanding of population-specific risk factors that may play a role in patients' lives. Learning more about any climate-sensitive health conditions (eg, history of reactions to aeroallergens, previous episodes of heat illness), social factors that contribute to climate resilience (eg, housing instability, access to heating and cooling, food security), and residence in high-risk geographic areas (eg, locations experiencing increasingly frequent or severe weather events, ambient air pollution, high levels of ultraviolet (UV) exposure, or all of these) is particularly important. Suggestions for specific messaging can be found in **Table 2**.

- *First*, solicit any clear exacerbating factors related to environmental exposures and determine if the patient may have been exposed to any recent extreme weather events. Ask parents/guardians open-ended questions to discuss whether they have noticed any clear exacerbating factors related to their child's condition. For example, "Have there been recent changes in environmental conditions?" or "Do symptoms worsen with outdoor exposure or did they newly develop after outdoor trips?" If weather events such as heat waves, wildfires, or hurricanes have recently occurred, ask about potential exposures to temperature changes, smoke, standing water, zoonotic disease vectors, and any environmental pollutants, as well as any physical trauma or signs of psychosocial stress.

- *Second*, elicit information about environmental exposures and symptoms of climate-sensitive conditions as you gather the patient's past medical history. Note that the changing climate is altering the distribution of primary outdoor allergens such as grasses, trees, weeds, fungal spores, and insects, as well as the intensity, seasonality, and duration of pollen seasons.[2,33] Indoor exposures include mold, pesticides, tobacco smoke, and animal dander. Common climate-sensitive conditions in pediatric populations include heat illness; aeroallergen-related disorders such as allergic rhinitis, conjunctivitis, and asthma; and respiratory diseases that may be worsened by chronic exposure to ambient air pollution. Many of these pollutants are combustion product irritants such as carbon dioxide, volatile organic compounds, lead, nitrogen dioxide, and sulfur dioxide. If flares of contact dermatitis, atopic dermatitis, acute urticaria, or other inflammatory dermatoses tend to co-occur with these types of exposures, the patient may be at higher risk of climate-sensitive health impacts now and in the future.

- *Third*, include details regarding the patient's long-term climate environment as part of their social history. For example, residential moves can result in temperature, humidity, and UV exposure changes that have implications for dermatologic diseases. Geographic location can also be an important determinant of weather-related risk; coastal communities face more frequent and severe floods, whereas those in the Western United States are subject to drought and wildfires. Housing stability can be particularly important to building climate resilience and is often first-line

Table 2
Examples of climate messaging in the pediatric dermatology encounter

Types of Health Risk	Dermatologic Disease Examples	Predisposing Factors	Sample Script
Vector-borne, zoonotic, and other infectious diseases	Cutaneous leishmaniasis, Lyme disease, hand-foot-and-mouth disease, dengue, Zika virus disease, coccidioidomycosis, chikungunya, Chagas disease, dermatophyte infections	• Recent relocation • Increased temperatures and precipitation[34] • Recent flooding • Frequent droughts[34] • Climate migration • Time outdoors • Housing insecurity	"The habitats and travel patterns of mosquitoes and other insects that carry disease are changing, which means we're starting to see infections in our area that used to only occur in tropical regions. Let's talk about what you should look out for when your child is outdoors."
Inflammatory dermatoses and related disease flares	Atopic dermatitis, psoriasis, urticaria, contact dermatitis, lichen planus, cheilitis	• Higher temperatures and increased sunlight[35] • Ozone exposures • Longer and more intense pollen seasons • Increased air pollution • Increased precipitation and mold spores[35] • Frequent droughts[35] • Time outdoors	"The intensity and length of pollen seasons has recently increased, which increased allergic exposures and can make skin diseases like atopic dermatitis worse. Let's talk about ways we can protect your child against allergens and free resources such as the Air Quality Index monitor."
Heat-related illnesses	Heat rash, miliaria, prickly heat	• Recent wildfires • Increasing temperatures and time outdoors • High physical activity levels • Social isolation • Housing insecurity • Lack of access to air conditioning • Urban environment	"Our area is experiencing more hot days because of environmental changes, and the heat can be especially tough on children who are active or outdoors a lot. Let's discuss ways that you can be prepared to keep your child cool and options for making sure that they get breaks from the heat."
Ozone/UV-related disease	Skin cancers, photodamage, phytophotodermatitis	• Increased temperatures and sun exposure • Other ozone exposures	"Changing climate patterns have increased our exposure to harmful UV rays that can cause skin cancer. Let's talk about a sun safety plan for your child."

(continued on next page)

Table 2
(continued)

Types of Health Risk	Dermatologic Disease Examples	Predisposing Factors	Sample Script
Physical trauma and crowding	Skin and soft tissue injuries, lice and scabies infestations	• Extreme weather events, especially hurricanes, that are increasing in severity and/or frequency • Local infrastructure damage • Climate migration • Transportation insecurity	"Global weather changes are causing more people to have to move from their homes into facilities with other families. Let's talk about any crowding you might be experiencing and some housing resources that may help."
Nutritional deficiency	Kwashiorkor, marasmus, scurvy, xerosis/pruritus, telogen effluvium, glossitis, angular cheilitis, pellagra, acrocyanosis, gingivitis	• Recent drought • Extreme weather events • Disruptions in local crop yields • Food insecurity • Poverty	"More frequent droughts and wildfires in our area that have driven down crop production and destroyed animals we rely on for food. Let's go over some resources that can help your child meet their nutritional needs."
Waterborne disease	Melioidosis, leptospirosis, *Vibrio* wound infections and/or sepsis, cercarial dermatitis, sea bather's eruption	• Frequent extreme weather events, especially high precipitation, hurricanes, floods, and/or tornadoes[2] • Exposure to standing water • Droughts in areas with outdated water treatment systems[36] • Ocean/coastal ecosystem[36] • Nearby algal blooms • Contamination from runoff[36] • Water insecurity	"We've been experiencing more frequent flooding in our area. Let's talk about how to limit your child's exposure to standing water and ensure that your family has access to clean drinking water."
Psychological distress	Increased severity of itch perception, trichotillomania, compulsive skin picking, acne excoriée, flares of inflammatory dermatoses	• Extreme weather events • Climate migration • History of climate-related anxiety	"Over the past few years, the number of extreme weather events in our area has been increasing. This can be especially scary for young children, so let's talk about how we can support you and your child emotionally – do you know about the National Disaster Distress Helpline?"

protection against environmental exposures. Access to resilient heating, ventilation, and air-conditioning infrastructure can mitigate aeroallergen-related disease, as well as buffer increasingly large shifts in temperature. Air quality also varies significantly between urban, suburban, and rural areas, as does water quality, the density and distribution of zoonotic disease vectors, and the stability of food supply chains. Residents of areas more immediately affected by climate-related agriculture disruptions are potentially at higher risk of nutritional deficiencies and food insecurity. Keep in mind that changes in patients' geography or built environment can introduce new climate-sensitive exposures and contribute to the disease process.

- *Fourth*, ask about concerns regarding climate change in conversations about psychiatric health. Climate-related anxiety is increasingly common in younger patients, and those living in areas with repeated, long-term, or increasingly severe weather events may suffer from significant emotional distress.

Climate messaging and patient/guardian education

Sample scripts for climate messaging during the dermatologic encounter, some of which were inspired by a previous commentary,[22] are provided in **Table 1**. These examples can help frame educational discussions with patients and parents/guardians and should be augmented with additional information from local climate resources.

CLINICS CARE POINTS

- Children are at higher risk for serious morbidity from environmental exposures due to age-related physiology, long-term developmental impacts, and their unique reliance on caregivers.

- Experiences of climate change intersect with societal factors including systemic racism, poverty, and lack of access to health care.

- The distribution and presentation of many inflammatory, infectious, and sun-related dermatoses are affected by extreme weather events and chronic environmental exposures.

- Targeted risk communication, motivational interviewing, and storytelling are discussion strategies that can be used to frame climate discussions with parents/guardians during the clinical encounter (see **Table 1**).

- Climate-related risk factors for dermatologic conditions can be elicited as part of the medical and social history. Examples of these predisposing factors include recent geographic changes, exposure to weather events, local infrastructure disruptions, and higher surface temperatures, which may predispose infectious dermatoses, inflammatory disease exacerbations, and heat-related illnesses, among other conditions (see **Table 2**).

SUMMARY

Pediatric dermatologists have a unique opportunity to protect the welfare of children given our changing climate. By providing concrete and actionable information during the clinical encounter, providers can reduce climate-related anxiety and empower families to best protect the health and safety of their loved ones. Given the fatal consequences of misinformation, as evidenced during the COVID-19 pandemic, it is critical that dermatologists provide credible and potentially lifesaving information regarding climate change, which represents one of the most significant threats to pediatric—and human—health.

DISCLOSURE

The authors have nothing to disclose.

REFERENCES

1. Sun M, Rosenbach M. The climate emergency: why should dermatologists care and how can they act? Br J Dermatol 2021;184(3):546–7.
2. Kaffenberger BH, Shetlar D, Norton SA, et al. The effect of climate change on skin disease in North America. J Am Acad Dermatol 2017;76(1):140–7.
3. Philipsborn RP, Chan K. Climate change and global child health. Pediatrics 2018;141(6):e20173774.
4. Watts N, Amann M, Arnell N, et al. The 2019 report of the lancet countdown on health and climate change: ensuring that the health of a child born today is not defined by a changing climate. Lancet 2019; 394(10211):1836–78.
5. Carlton EJ, Woster AP, DeWitt P, et al. A systematic review and meta-analysis of ambient temperature and diarrhoeal diseases. Int J Epidemiol 2016; 45(1):117–30.
6. Lelieveld J, Pozzer A, Pöschl U, et al. Loss of life expectancy from air pollution compared to other risk factors: a worldwide perspective. Cardiovasc Res 2020;116(11):1910–7.
7. Reid CE, Considine EM, Watson GL, et al. Associations between respiratory health and ozone and fine

particulate matter during a wildfire event. Environ Int 2019;129:291–8.

8. Shao J, Zosky GR, Wheeler AJ, et al. Exposure to air pollution during the first 1000 days of life and subsequent health service and medication usage in children. Environ Pollut 2020;256:113340.

9. Nguyen GH, Andersen LK, Davis MDP. Climate change and atopic dermatitis: is there a link? Int J Dermatol 2019;58(3):279–82.

10. Steinhoff M, Suárez AL, Feramisco JD, et al. Psychoneuroimmunology of psychological stress and atopic dermatitis: pathophysiologic and therapeutic updates. Acta Derm Venereol 2012;92(1):7–15.

11. Stewart TJ, Tong W, Whitfeld MJ. The associations between psychological stress and psoriasis: a systematic review. Int J Dermatol 2018;57(11):1275–82.

12. Simons RE, Zevy DL, Jafferany M. Psychodermatology of vitiligo: psychological impact and consequences. Dermatol Ther 2020;33(3):e13418.

13. Katsarou-Katsari A, Singh LK, Theoharides TC. Alopecia areata and affected skin CRH receptor upregulation induced by acute emotional stress. Dermatology 2001;203(2):157–61.

14. Lewis KLM, Avery CW, Reidmiller DR. Fourth national climate assessment, volume II: impacts, risks, and adaptation in the United States. U.S. Global Change Research Program; 2018.

15. Davies IP, Haugo RD, Robertson JC, et al. The unequal vulnerability of communities of color to wildfire. PLoS One 2018;13(11):e0205825.

16. Tessum CW, Apte JS, Goodkind AL, et al. Inequity in consumption of goods and services adds to racial-ethnic disparities in air pollution exposure. Proc Natl Acad Sci U S A 2019;116(13):6001–6.

17. National Low Income Housing Coalition. Annu Rep. 2018.

18. DeBono R, Vincenti K, Calleja N. Risk communication: climate change as a human-health threat, a survey of public perceptions in Malta. Eur J Public Health 2012;22(1):144–9.

19. Kelley JM, Kraft-Todd G, Schapira L, et al. The influence of the patient-clinician relationship on healthcare outcomes: a systematic review and meta-analysis of randomized controlled trials. PLoS One 2014;9(4):e94207.

20. Mabon L. Making climate information services accessible to communities: what can we learn from environmental risk communication research? Urban Clim 2020;31:100537.

21. MacIntyre E, Khanna S, Darychuk A, et al. Evidence synthesis - Evaluating risk communication during extreme weather and climate change: a scoping review. Health Promot Chronic Dis Prev Can 2019; 39(4):142–56.

22. Senay E, Sarfaty M, Rice MB. Strategies for clinical discussions about climate change. Ann Intern Med 2020;174(3):417–8.

23. Dressler C, Lambert J, Grine L, et al. Therapeutic patient education and self-management support for patients with psoriasis - a systematic review. J Dtsch Dermatol Ges 2019;17(7):685–95.

24. Chisholm A, Nelson PA, Pearce CJ, et al. Motivational interviewing-based training enhances clinicians' skills and knowledge in psoriasis: findings from the Pso Well(®) study. Br J Dermatol 2017;176(3):677–86.

25. Lusilla-Palacios P, Masferrer E. Motivational interviewing in dermatology. Actas Dermosifiliogr 2016; 107(8):627–30.

26. Moezzi M, Janda KB, Rotmann S. Using stories, narratives, and storytelling in energy and climate change research. Energy Res Soc Sci 2017;31:1–10.

27. Dahlstrom MF. Using narratives and storytelling to communicate science with nonexpert audiences. Proc Natl Acad Sci U S A 2014;111(Supplement 4):13614–20.

28. Paschen J-A, Ison R. Narrative research in climate change adaptation—Exploring a complementary paradigm for research and governance. Res Policy 2014;43(6):1083–92.

29. Gross L. Confronting climate change in the age of denial. Plos Biol 2018;16(10):e3000033.

30. Brown P. Narrative: an ontology, epistemology and methodology for pro-environmental psychology research. Energy Res Soc Sci 2017;31:215–22.

31. Vulturius G, André K, Swartling ÅG, et al. Does climate change communication matter for individual engagement with adaptation? insights from forest owners in Sweden. Environ Manage 2020;65(2): 190–202.

32. Otto D. Lived experience of climate change - A digital storytelling approach. Int J Glob Warming 2017; 12:331.

33. Coates PS, Ricca MA, Prochazka BG, et al. Wildfire, climate, and invasive grass interactions negatively impact an indicator species by reshaping sagebrush ecosystems. Proc Natl Acad Sci U S A 2016;113(45):12745–50.

34. Vectorborne and zoonotic diseases. National institute of environmental health sciences. National Institutes of Health; 2018. Available at: https://www.niehs.nih.gov/ research/programs/climatechange/health_impacts/ vectorborne/index.cfm. Accessed April 1, 2020.

35. Asthma, respiratory allergies and airway diseases. National Institute of Environmental Health Sciences: National Institutes of Health; 2017. Available at: https://www.niehs.nih.gov/research/programs/ climatechange/health_impacts/asthma/index.cfm. Accessed April 1, 2020.

36. Waterborne diseases. National institute of environmental health sciences. National Institutes of Health; 2017. Available at: https://www.niehs.nih.gov/ research/programs/climatechange/health_impacts/ waterborne_diseases/index.cfm. Accessed April 1, 2020.

Moving?

Make sure your subscription moves with you!

To notify us of your new address, find your **Clinics Account Number** (located on your mailing label above your name), and contact customer service at:

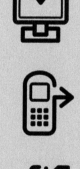

Email: journalscustomerservice-usa@elsevier.com

800-654-2452 (subscribers in the U.S. & Canada)
314-447-8871 (subscribers outside of the U.S. & Canada)

Fax number: 314-447-8029

Elsevier Health Sciences Division
Subscription Customer Service
3251 Riverport Lane
Maryland Heights, MO 63043

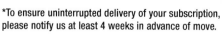

ELSEVIER

Printed and bound by CPI Group (UK) Ltd, Croydon, CR0 4YY

11/05/2025

01866591-0001